Pilates
Workbook

Pilates Workbook

Illustrated step-by-step guide to matwork techniques

MICHAEL KING

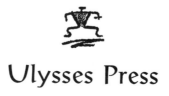

Ulysses Press

Published in the United States by
Ulysses Press
P.O. Box 3440
Berkeley, CA 94703
www.ulyssespress.com

First published as *Pure Pilates* in 2000 by Mitchell Beazley
an imprint of Octopus Publishing Group Ltd

Library of Congress Card Number 2001091809
ISBN 1-56975-276-1

Printed in Canada by Transcontinental Printing

10 9 8 7 6

Interior Design	Kenny Grant
Cover Design	Sarah Levin
Photography	Ruth Jenkinson
Models	Beth Caterer
	Simon Spalding

Distributed in the United States by Publishers Group West

Please Note
This book has been written and published strictly for
informational purposes, and in no way should be used as a
substitute for consultation with health care professionals. You
should not consider educational material herein to be the
practice of medicine or to replace consultation with a physician
or other medical practitioner. The author and publisher are
providing you with information in this work so that you can
have the knowledge and can choose, at your own risk, to act
on that knowledge. The author and publisher also urge all
readers to be aware of their health status and to consult health
care professionals before beginning any health program,
including changes in dietary habits.

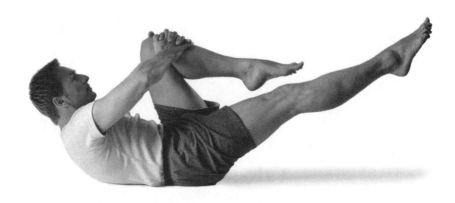

contents

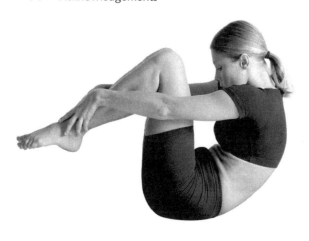

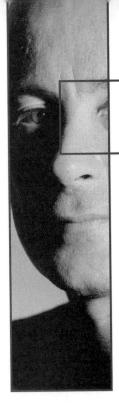

introduction

Pilates is not just a series of exercises, it is a conceptual approach to movement. It will change not only the way you look, but how you feel and think. The technique can be taught in different ways—for strength or relaxation. In Pilates Workbook we aim for a balance of both.

Twenty-two years ago I came across Pilates as a dancer at the London School of Contemporary Dance. Though it was part of our daily training, I didn't really understand the importance of it. It wasn't until I began practicing Pilates to repair a back injury that I really began to appreciate its power and effectiveness. I loved what it did to heal my body. I was so inspired by the method, I went on to train with Alan Herdman, the first teacher to bring Pilates from America to Britain.

In 1982 I opened my own studio, Body Control, in connection with the newly formed Pineapple Dance Studios in Covent Garden. Two years later I was offered a job in Texas to run the Pilates studio at the Houston Ballet Company, which was set up both for dancers and outside patrons. (During this time I also trained to teach the new Fonda-established aerobics.) I have taught Pilates ever since.

It is so exciting to see the recent boom in popularity that Pilates has enjoyed. From both the experience of my own back injury and my extensive work within the fitness world, I have come to appreciate the true value and significance of the technique. I used to think that becoming hunched up was an inevitable part of the aging process. I now see that how we treat our bodies from day to day can affect how we feel and look as we get older.

My goal is to pass on the information and knowledge that I have picked up over the years and to share the secrets I've found that make this work successful. Pilates is a very varied technique and can be taught in many formats and styles. I believe that through practicing pure Pilates we can all achieve better balance, gain leaner bodies and feel more poised and less stressed. Always remember that it just as crucial to master the

vital elements behind the technique as it is to simply perform the movements. Pilates is not just a series of physical exercises but a concept-based routine that will challenge old assumptions. Pilates has been called a "thinking way of moving." It involves making a commitment to yourself, your body and your well-being. You can know all the movements and still not properly appreciate Pilates.

The total concept also involves getting enough sleep, eating right and continuing your usual fitness program. Through the years I've combined my early Pilates training with regular fitness training. Pilates is not an "instead of" but an "as well as." In other words, it doesn't replace your current fitness programs but is a valuable and necessary addition.

I know that you will find Pilates to be as empowering for you as it has been for me.

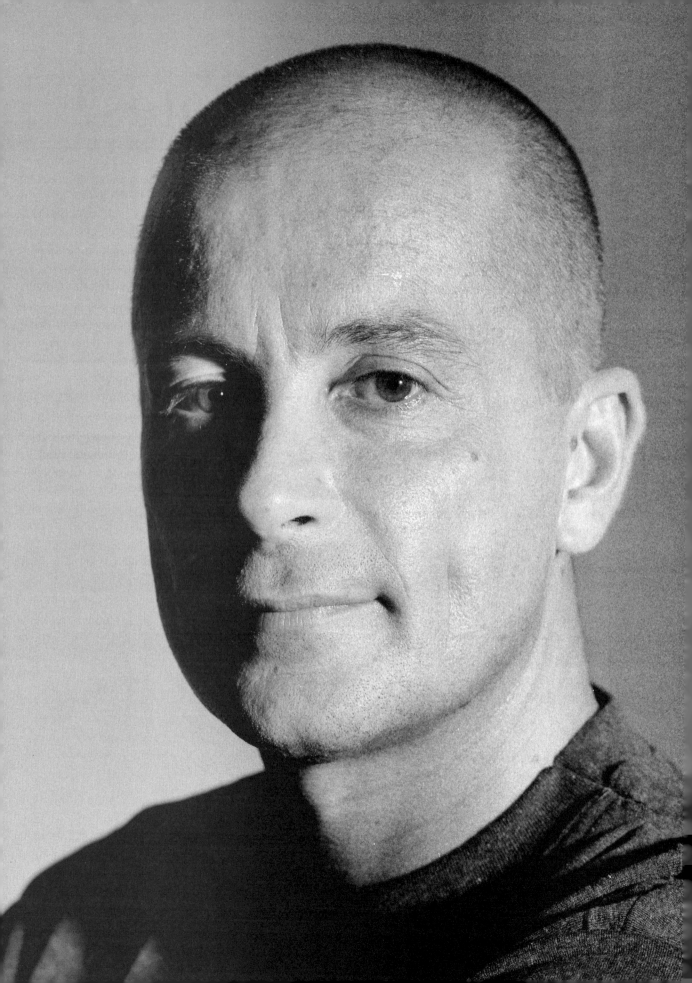

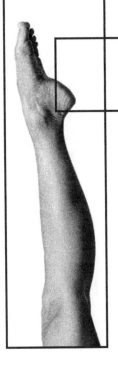

what is pilates?

Pilates offers a different way of thinking about your body. Through practicing the movements, you will become more self-aware and better able to take control of your body and your life. Although the technique may at times take you outside your comfort zone, the benefits of this are that you begin to understand and appreciate not only your strengths, but also your weaknesses.

At this, the beginning of a new millennium, there has been a renewed interest in exercise techniques that also acknowledge the power of the mind. Pilates, like Feldenkrais, the Alexander technique and yoga, fall under this mind–body umbrella. All these techniques offer alternative philosophies to conventional thinking about health and fitness.

Mind and movement
Pilates is named after its inventor, Joseph Pilates, who formulated the exercises in the 1920s. There are 34 original Pilates movements. As well as matwork, there are also equipment-based routines. These pieces of equipment, devised by Joseph Pilates himself, have strange and wonderful names such as The Wunda Chair, The Cadillac and the Pedi-Pul. In a traditional Pilates studio you work half the session on the equipment and the other half performing

matwork exercises. Each offers different benefits. If you can get to a Pilates studio, you will find this out for yourself: working on equipment is great. Alternatively, if this is impossible, the matwork exercises provide an extremely thorough program in the convenience of your own home.

Beauty and benefit
Pilates has been around for the last seventy years but has recently drawn much media coverage. Many Hollywood stars have given the technique their endorsement. Madonna, for example, affirmed that Pilates is the only way to exercise. As a result of such public praise, Pilates is no longer an exclusive secret of the rich and famous. What once might have seemed like a strange cult activity is now a popular class in health clubs the world over. While some people become interested in Pilates for its cosmetic body-

Celebrity endorsement
Pilates has always attracted a star following. Initially Lauren Bacall and Gregory Peck were interested in the technique. Now a whole new generation has embraced Pilates, including actress Jodie Foster, dancer Wayne Sleep, tennis player Pat Cash and pop icon Madonna.

sculpting effects, others come to it through referrals by their physiotherapist or medical practitioner. In particular, Pilates has been the first exercise choice for many, like myself, who have injured their backs. I see Pilates as an excellent preventative technique that will strengthen your body against potential injury. It cannot, however, act as a replacement for medical advice. If you have a physical problem, find out what is going on before attempting the Pilates movements. Specific problems should be addressed by a qualified therapist.

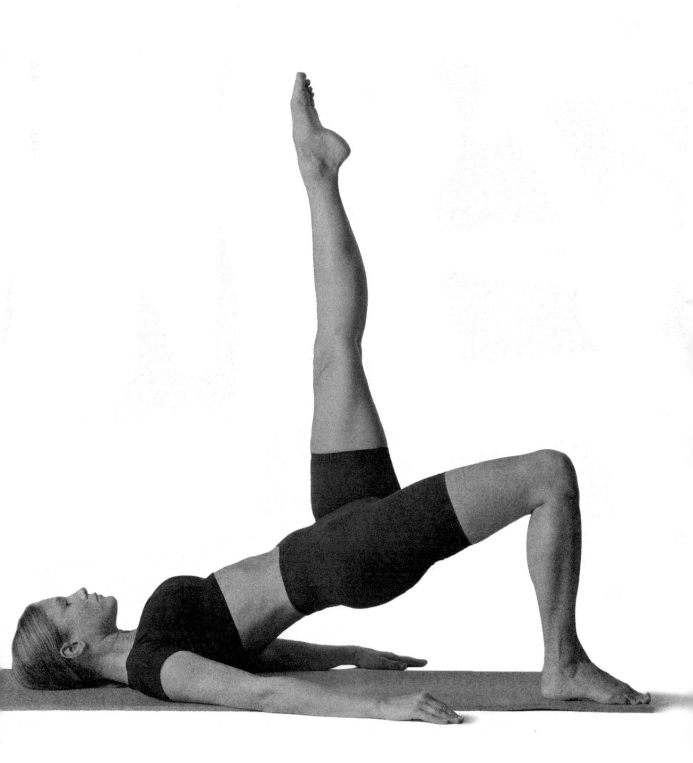

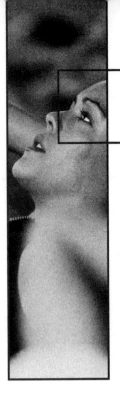

why pilates?

Pilates is unique in that it will systematically exercise all the muscle groups in your body, the weak as well as the strong. It combines the focus on suppleness that you find in yoga with the emphasis on strength building found in the gym. In this way, it aims to create balance and natural poise, taking into consideration all the factors involved in the maintenance of a healthy body.

People often wonder how Pilates exercises can change body shape. The secret is simple. Pilates movements gently stretch the muscles, pulling them into leaner and longer shapes. It might help if I explain what I mean by the term "longer." Bodybuilders increase their muscle bulk by overloading muscles, tearing fibers and causing them to rebuild. In the process the muscle becomes shorter and thicker. Pilates is different because it does exactly the opposite. It works by continually stretching your limbs and torso, ensuring muscles become longer and leaner rather than shorter and thicker.

New thinking

It is now recognized that the regular fitness regimes we have been doing for so many years are not so much wrong as incomplete. We have made exercise very safe: people no longer injure themselves in the gym, but do pull muscles at home or work when they lift something heavy out of a car or pick up their small child. This is because standard exercise does not prepare the body for these activities. Traditionally, exercise and strength training has compartmentalized the body, training individual body parts, such as the bicep in a bicep curl or the quadricep in a leg extension. But we have not trained our body parts to work together, in synergy.

United we stand

Think of an orchestra rehearsing; the brass section might practice in one room and the strings rehearse in another. The symphony only comes together when all parts of the orchestra play together. Standard exercise keeps sections of the orchestra practicing separately. While each section may be strong and technically

Lines of symmetry

The body is built along lines of symmetry and every exertion is subject to checks and balances. Lift your left arm up until it is horizontal and hold it there. Put your other hand to the right-hand side of your back. You should be able to feel the muscles in your back clenching.

skilled, they still need to rehearse together in order to make music and achieve complete balance.

Functional fitness

"Functional fitness" is a hot topic today. Magazines are full of articles on the subject. But what does it mean? Let me explain by going back to the gym to look at the regular seated bench press. A seated bench press involves sitting on the equipment and pushing the weight in front of you. On a good day you might be able to push 40, 50, possibly 60 pounds. However, if you were to

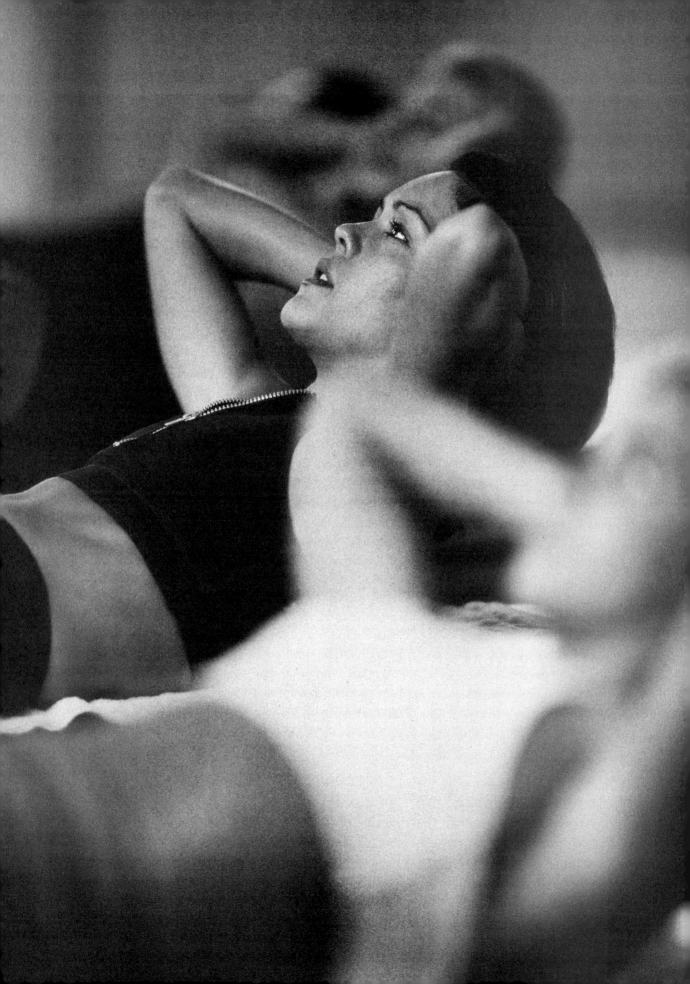

move one inch forward of the back support, you would only be able to push around a third of the weight. Here, without the support of the chair behind you, you can measure the true extent of your functional strength.

Sitting up and listening

I have come to realize the extent to which the shape of our bodies reflects our day-to-day activities. Whether we are aware of it or not, we literally shape ourselves. Those with the best posture in the world are the traditional Japanese. Why? They have no backs to their chairs. Here in the Western world we have made life very comfortable by designing the most supportive chair, car and airline seat. We do not ask much of the body in daily activities. In the morning we go from sitting behind our breakfast table, to sitting behind our steering wheel, to sitting behind our desk, to sitting behind our lunch table. Then it is back to the desk, home in the car again, sitting in front of the TV, back to bed. Three times a week we might go to the gym and do sit-ups hoping this will bring balance to our lives. Is it any surprise that 80% of us will experience back pain in our lives?

Train for life

Modern living has made life so easy that we don't ask our backs to work. Sadly, in contemporary Japan, the young Japanese now have the same postural problems that we suffer. We talk about going to the gym to train, but we are constantly training our bodies to behave in other ways during the remaining hours of the day when we are not at the gym.

With modern life leaving so little room for an integrated program of exercise, it is no wonder that there has been a significant movement in recent years towards mind and body techniques. Only these disciplines offer the opportunity of using our bodies in a complete way. We exercise to improve our "quality of life." Yet what does this mean? It means we want our daily lives to be improved and enriched. We want to be able, for example, to carry the shopping, lift a child, move a wardrobe or push a car if it breaks down. It is these kinds of daily activity that demand functional strength.

Professional posture

Functional exercises are exercises designed to be appropriate to the needs of everyday living. Many of the people who come to my class at lunchtime sit behind a desk all day long. As a Pilates instructor I train them to sit (strengthening their core stability) since they are "professional sitters." There is little purpose in focusing on the biggest bicep or the strongest leg. It is not that these things are not important and should not be worked on, but my priority has to be on strengthening their body for the longest activity of the day. Pilates will develop the areas that need attention and build strength in our weakest areas. Building strength in the abdomen is vital to most daily activities as it is this area which provides core stability.

Symmetry and synergy

I like to compare using the body to putting up a tent. Our movements are comprised of a series of checks and balances; exertion on the right side of the body will be compensated for on the left. For a tent to be secure there has to be an equal amount of tension on both front and back ropes. If the tension is too tight, the ropes are in danger of snapping and there is no flexibility against winds. If we always pull on one side, our "tent" of muscles will veer out of balance. If we only train our abdominals and not our back, then we are pulling on just one section of our "tent strings." Only when there is equal tension between front and back, our right sides and our left, can true stability and balance be achieved.

An integrated approach

Our bodies demand an integrated approach whereby no single muscle is developed at the expense of another. The body is built on lines of symmetry and the Pilates exercise technique acknowledges and exploits this fact. The daily habits of our lives often mitigate against an integrated approach and we find ourselves leading sedentary working lives in offices where there is little scope for using our full physical potential. Medical conditions such as "repetitive strain" can result. Pilates can redress the balance and help us to become more aware of what we unconsciously do to our bodies. Through self-awareness we can identify and alter our bad habits.

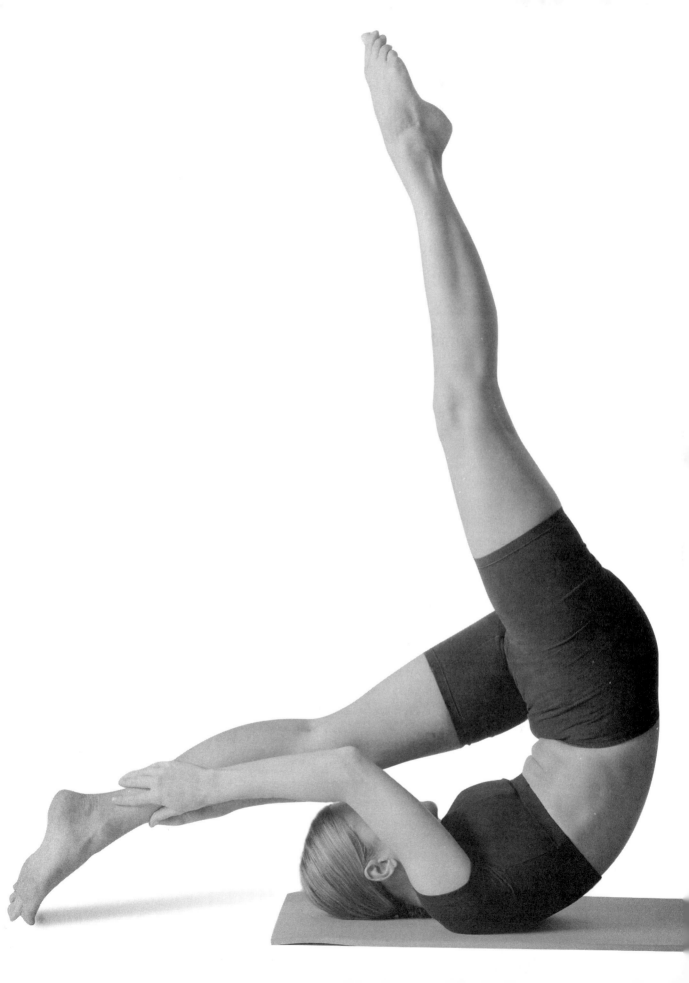

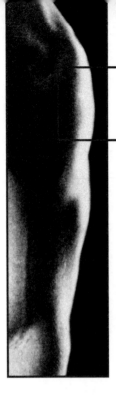

why pure pilates?

The original, authentic matwork exercises, as devised by Joseph Pilates, are more taxing than the simplified moves advocated by many teachers. You will have to work up to pure Pilates movements gradually, using the easier alternatives we offer. But if you want real results, original is best.

Pilates offers a whole-body workout that challenges your body like no other exercise. When Joseph Pilates devised the original matwork exercises, he did not intend to spare us any effort. Even the fittest of athletes will find some of the original moves very difficult to complete, simply because they require the control and coordination of muscles that few of us are accustomed to using.

Easing your way in

In order to make life easier for beginners, many teachers have devised diluted versions of the movements. There is a real place for this. Not everybody can go straight to the crab or the leg pull without gradually easing the muscles into use. This is why I have listed alternative moves alongside all the main moves in the book—to allow you to begin on an easier version. There may be some people for whom physical constraints or medical conditions mean that they cannot progress onto pure Pilates. This is fine. Part of Pilates is knowing your limits and working within them. However, if you are fairly fit and flexible, you will find that you can move on to the advanced exercises more quickly. Joseph Pilates developed the movements to challenge muscles, knowing that for you, as for him, it would lead to perfect toning. These exercises are designed to elongate and stretch the muscles in order to create a sleek and leaner look.

Pure is best

The pure forms of the movements give you the best results as they are more intense. For this reason I have presented the pure form first and the alternatives afterwards. I believe it is always good to see what you are aiming for. Although there is no one single right or wrong way to teach or practice

Who's right or wrong?

By knowing pure Pilates you'll have a reference point to understand the variations on the movements taught by different instructors. Variations offer a range of distinct effects and benefits. The specialist knowledge and background of the instructors determines how they interpret the Pilates movements. It is a testament to the effectiveness of the original technique that so many others have learnt from it and gone on to devise their own programs.

Pilates, it is these pure movements that have best stood the test of time. If we are physically capable, we should aspire to achieve the original moves. Attaining good results will also involve understanding the principles, the vital elements that make the discipline what it is. In this book we have presented these elements one by one so that you can understand the full meaning and benefits of Pilates matwork.

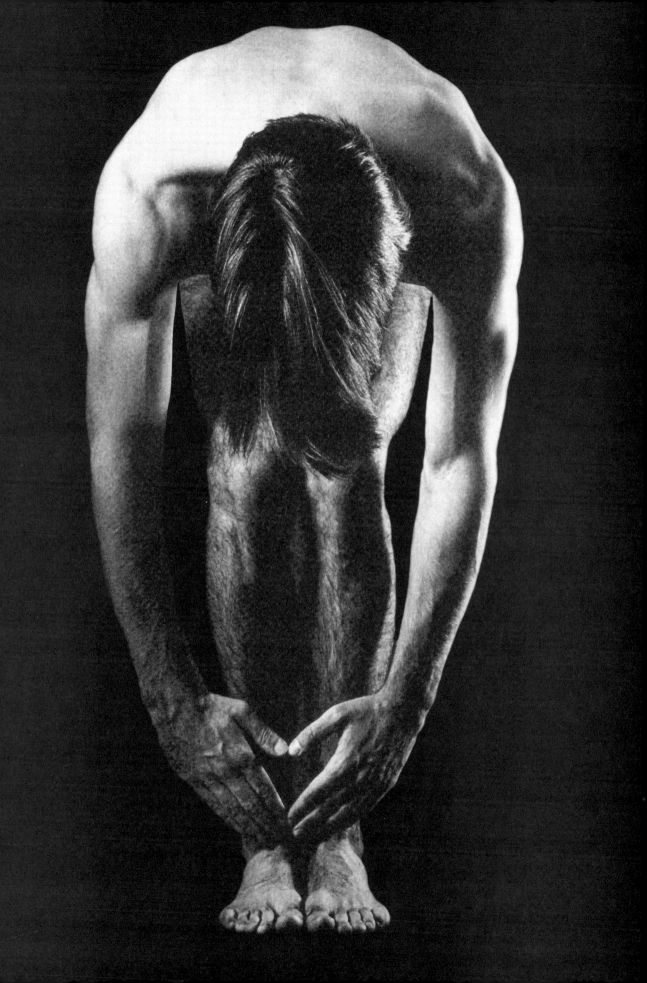

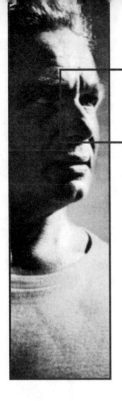

man and mentor

Prone to childhood illness, Joseph Pilates refused to let poor physical health cloud his future. Determined to fulfil his potential, he studied bodybuilding, gymnastics, boxing and diving until he had mastered them all. After years of study, he developed an approach to fitness that would change the way people viewed physical exercise. This is his intriguing story.

Joseph Humbertus Pilates was born near Dussledorf, Germany, in 1880. He suffered from a range of debilitating conditions throughout his childhood including rickets, asthma and rheumatic fever. Determined to overcome his poor physical health, he devoted himself to the task of becoming as fit and strong as was humanly possible. This determination was characteristic of Pilates' spirited and forceful personality. His early fierce reaction to illness would inform all his future enterprises.

Excelling in fitness

In his youth Pilates studied and became proficient at numerous sports and fitness activities, including skiing, gymnastics, diving and bodybuilding. By the time he was 14 years old, he was in such good shape that he was able to work as a model for anatomical charts. In 1912, Pilates moved from Germany to England where he earned a living in a wide variety of jobs that required him to be in peak physical condition. He worked as a boxer, circus performer and a self-defence trainer of English detectives.

Exercise innovator

When World War I broke out Pilates was interned because of his nationality. He was held in camps in Lancaster and the Isle of Man. While there he acted as a physician to the other men. It seemed a natural step for him eventually to take responsibility for the health of the other interns and he began training them in physical fitness. It was then that he first improvised making fitness equipment, removing the springs from the beds and attaching them to the walls above the beds so that patients could exercise while lying down. After the war, Pilates continued his fitness programs back in Germany, in Hamburg, where he worked with the police force before being drafted into the army. By 1926, disenchanted with Germany, he decided to move to America. On the ship to New York he met a nurse called Clara, the woman he was to later marry.

Guru to dancers

Soon after arriving in New York, Pilates set up his first exercise studio at 939 Eighth Avenue. Though little is known about the early years of his business, by the 1940s Joe had achieved a certain amount of notoriety amongst the city's dance community. "At some time or other," reported *Dance Magazine* in its February 1956 issue, "virtually every dancer in New York had meekly submitted to the spirited instruction of Joe Pilates." By the early 1960s, Pilates could count many of New York's finest dancers among his clients. George Balanchine, one of ballet's foremost choreographers and

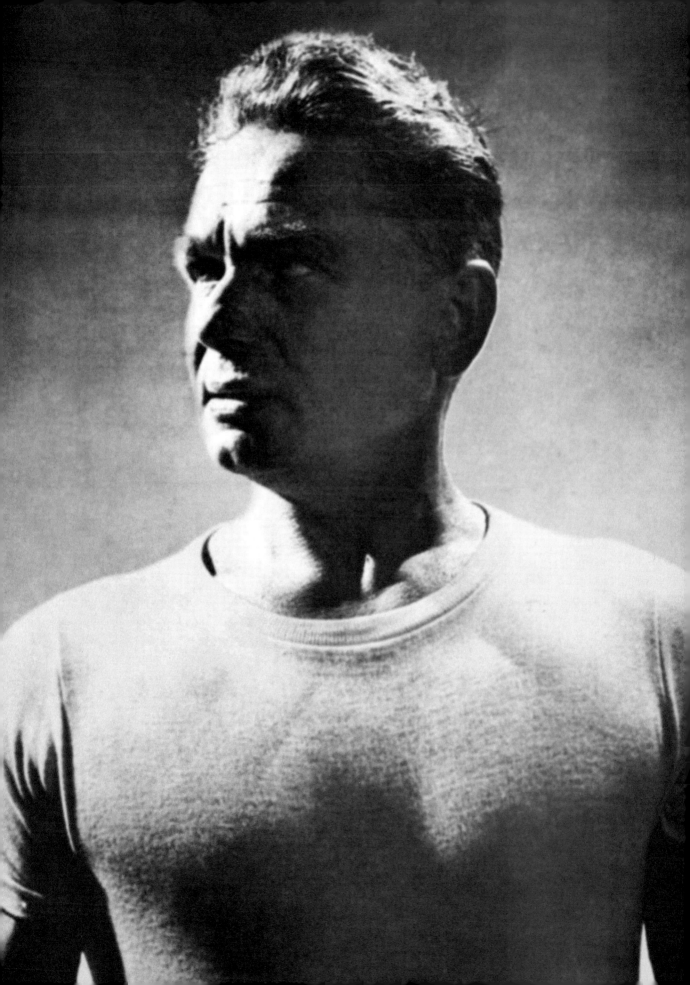

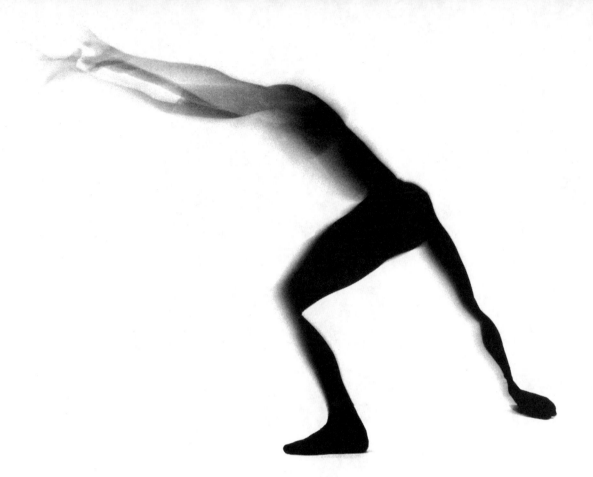

co-founder of the New York City Ballet, worked out "at Joe's," as he called it, and also invited Pilates to instruct the young dancers of his acclaimed ballet company. "Pilates," as it was now becoming known, was catching on and becoming very popular outside New York City as well. As the *New York Herald Tribune* noted in 1964, "In dance classes around the United States, hundreds of young students limber up daily with an exercise they know as a Pilates, without knowing that the word has a capital P, and a living, right-breathing namesake."

The next generation
Just two of Joe's students, Carola Trier and Bob Seed, are known to have opened their own Pilates studios while Joe was still living.

Trier had an extensive dance background. She had found her way to the United States after escaping being sent to a Nazi concentration camp in France by becoming a contortionist in a circus show. She discovered Pilates in 1940, when a non-stage injury effectively curtailed her performing career as a dancer. Joe Pilates assisted Trier in opening her own studio in the late 1950s. Bob Seed was another story. A former male nurse turned Pilates enthusiast, Seed opened his own studio across the street from Joe's. He allegedly tried poaching some of Joe's clients by opening his studio in the early morning. It was rumored that, as a result of this betrayal, Joe visited Seed with a gun and warned him to get out of town. Seed promptly left.

The legacy
When Joe passed away in 1967, he was 87 years old. He left no will and had designated no successor to carry on the Pilates exercise work. Nevertheless, due to the popularity and effectiveness of the technique, his work was destined to continue.

Clara, Joe's wife, continued to operate what was already known as the Pilates Studio in New York and Romana Kryzanowska, a former student who had been instructed by Pilates in the 1940s, became its director in the 1970s.

Other students of Pilates went on to open their own studios. Ron Fletcher, a dancer who trained under Martha Graham, the central figure of the modern dance movement, studied and consulted with Joe from the 1940s in connection with a chronic knee ailment. Fletcher eventually opened his own Pilates studio in Los Angeles in 1970, where he attracted many of Hollywood's brightest stars. Clara was particularly enamored with Ron and gave her blessing for him to carry on the Pilates work and name.

Like Carola Trier, Fletcher brought numerous innovations and advancements to the Pilates technique. His evolving variations on Pilates were inspired both by his years in modern dance and by another mentor, ballet instructor Yeichi Nimura.

Kathy Grant and Lolita San Miguel were also students of Joe who went on to become teachers. Grant took over the direction at the Bendel's studio in 1972, while San Miguel went on to teach Pilates at Ballet Concierto de Puerto Rica in San Juan, Puerto Rico. In 1967, just before Joe's death, both Grant and San Miguel were awarded degrees by the State University of New York to teach Pilates. These two are believed to be the only Pilates practitioners ever to be certified officially by Joe himself.

His wider influence

In order to formulate his ideas, Joseph Pilates studied across a range of different sports and exercise disciplines from both the East and the West. He was most influenced by the ideas of the ancient Greeks and often quoted the admonition that in life we should abide by the rule "Not too little, not too much." He was one of the first people to promote an holistic approach. He looked to the natural world for clues about the human body and spent time, for example, looking closely at the movement of animals.

Joesph Pilates' ideas remain remarkably relevant. He blamed the "constant pushing, shoving, rushing, crowding and wild scrambling all so characteristic of our day" for many of our mental and bodily ills. "This too fast pace," he asserted, "is plainly reflected in our manner of standing, walking, sitting, eating and even talking and results in our nerves being on edge from morning to night." This applies more than ever to the busy, stressful lives we lead today.

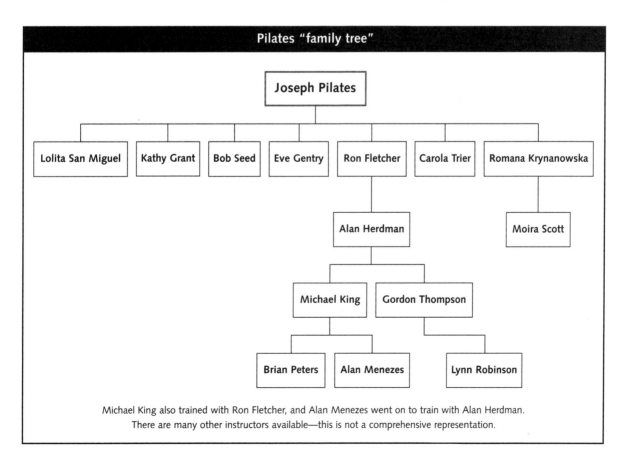

Pilates "family tree"

Joseph Pilates

Lolita San Miguel | Kathy Grant | Bob Seed | Eve Gentry | Ron Fletcher | Carola Trier | Romana Krynanowska

Alan Herdman

Moira Scott

Michael King | Gordon Thompson

Brian Peters | Alan Menezes | Lynn Robinson

Michael King also trained with Ron Fletcher, and Alan Menezes went on to train with Alan Herdman.
There are many other instructors available—this is not a comprehensive representation.

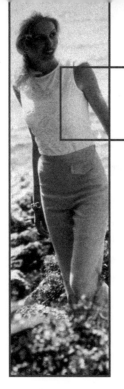

setting your goals

Whether your goal is to redefine your body shape, relieve stiffness or build strength, the first step is positive thinking. Pilates will change the shape of your body. I have seen it happen hundreds of times. I have also seen it help relieve back and hip pain and correct postural problems. Believe, practice, and watch it happen!

When I ask my new students what they want to get out of Pilates, the most common answer from the women is "I want to have a body like Madonna" while the men insist that they "want a six-pack stomach." Other goals most often mentioned include the relief of back pain or building strength.

Patience and practice

When I tell people that Pilates will change the shape of their bodies, the most commonly asked question is "How long will it take for me to see results?" "You'll see them instantly" is my reply. If you stand taller on your feet, pull your abdominals in tight and drop your shoulders, immediately you will look so much better! The question really should be "How long will it take for me to maintain this look without having to think about it?" The answer, realistically, is three to six months of regular practice.

Weighty matters

There is one frequently cited goal that is not achievable by Pilates alone: it will not help you lose weight. If you need to shed pounds, you should do some cardiovascular training 4–5 times per week (I find spin-cycle classes change the shape of body fat distribution most effectively) and follow a suitable nutritional program. There are many theories on nutrition, but I have found a food combining diet (separating consumption of carbohydrates and protein) and a reduction in fat intake works well for my clients.

Work on weaknesses

It is important to recognize where your strengths and weaknesses lie. By weakness I don't just mean lack of muscular strength. A tight, inflexible back is as problematic as a weak one. Because Pilates

exercises balance the body, different movements challenge us in different ways. I find that the movements my students least enjoy are usually the ones they cannot do very well. This often indicates a weakness. Instead of avoiding the exercises you enjoy the least, it is vital to persist.

A new shape

You might never look quite like Madonna, or have the perfect six-pack as a result of practicing Pilates, but good posture and longer, leaner muscles will make you look a new person. However, it will take time. We live in a society where we want everything "now." Instead, start thinking about your goals in the full knowledge that it is going to take a while for you to reap (and feel) the full benefits. I know it will happen, and I know that you will be delighted with the results.

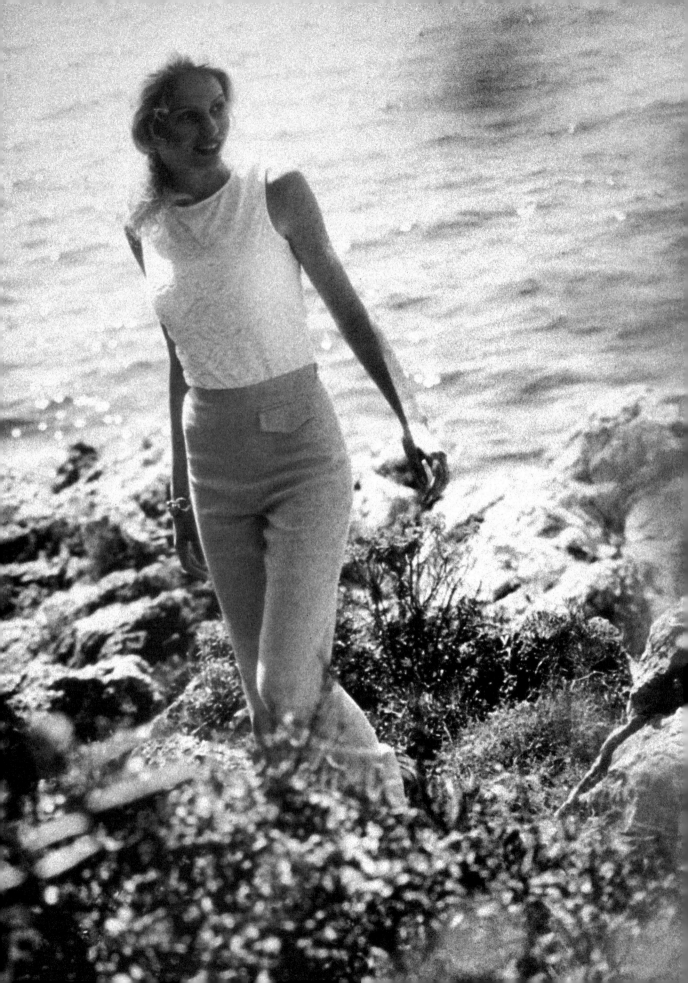

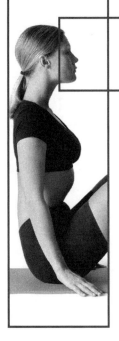

step-by-step plan

The charts on the following pages are designed to help you to put together your own exercise plan. Use them to combine different Pilates movements as you progress through levels of increasing difficulty and intensity. By following these guidelines you will gradually build up your strength and mobility in equal measure. Each exercise challenges muscle groups in a different way.

The charts on the following pages set out the combinations you need to follow in order to create your own Pilates routine. Always start with low intensity variations and only progress on to the harder variations once you feel happy and in control of your movement.

Patience pays

Pilates most benefits those who show the greatest patience. Do not be tempted to cheat and skip ahead to more advanced levels before you are ready. Even the fittest person should start at level one. Only in this way can you learn the base work so necessary to progress to harder exercises. You will know when you are ready to move on when you have fully mastered your breathing.

Do not rush

We live in a world which usually tells us that it is always better to exercise harder and faster to

achieve results. But with Pilates the opposite is true. Working slowly and correctly ensures the full use of all our muscles. The same principle is just as applicable in the gym. Slowly lifting up a light weight and carefully letting it down a number of times is far more productive than quickly jacking up a heavy weight and abruptly releasing it. Working slowly ensures you maximize your muscle effectiveness. Make sure you measure your own progress through the various levels by how thoroughly you are able to complete each movement.

Time for yourself

Before you begin, make sure you set a regular time and place for your workout. Some people prefer to exercise in the morning while others feel they are more flexible in the evenings. Always leave enough time to complete the program properly.

Cross-training

Just because you have started to exercise using the Pilates method, it does not mean that you have to give up on other sports and fitness programs. On the contrary, your Pilates program is best served when it is complemented by a form of cardiovascular exercise. Complete low-stress Pilates exercises alongside aerobic ones. You will find Pilates ideal for cross-training because it will correct any postural problem associated with other forms of repetitive exercise. Pilates embraces all the areas that make up a fully integrated approach to fitness; strength, flexibility, motor skills, coordination and relaxation.

Setting your pace

It might take a month or so to perfect each level although every individual's needs are different. Do things at the pace that feels right for you. You should not at any point experience any sudden or severe pain. If you start shaking or sweating, then you are pushing

Essential Exercise Chart

Page	Movement	Emphasis	Level 1	Level 2	Level 3	Level 4
54	PUSH-UP	Strength		o	o	o
56	SWIMMING	Strength	o	o	o	o
58	LEG PULL PRONE	Strength				o
60	ROLL-UP	Strength		o	o	o
62	ROLLING BACK	Mobility	o	o	o	o
63	ONE LEG CIRCLE	Mobility	o	o	o	o
64	THE HUNDRED	Strength	o	o	o	o
66	THE SEAL	Mobility			o	o
67	ONE LEG STRETCH	Strength			o	o
68	THE SAW	Mobility			o	o
69	SHOULDER BRIDGE PREP	Mobility	o	o	o	o
70	SIDE KICK	Strength			o	o
71	SPINE STRETCH	Mobility	o	o	o	o
72	SPINE TWIST	Mobility		o	o	o

things too far, too soon. As I have said before, expect your weaknesses to be revealed.

Starting off

Initially, each program should last around an hour. This amount of time allows for the completion of the first six movements. You should always split your moves into two halves, three for mobility and three for strength. In my classes, most people take around a month or so to master the exercises set out in level one. Aim to complete your exercise plan three or four times a week. After a few weeks, move onto the next level, adding two more strength and mobility moves each time. Introduce new movements slowly if you don't feel you can double up your exercise plan so quickly. Just how fast you progress through the program depends on a number of factors including how often you practice each week, for how long, and your physical condition at the start of the program. Do not despair if sometimes you feel less capable of achieving movements at the higher levels than at other times. It is normal for the body to feel more tired on some days than others. A small amount of regular exercise, correctly performed, is always better than erratic over-exertion. Joseph Pilates asserted that you should attempt at least ten minutes of Pilates a day "without fail." If you can only spare ten minutes, it is best to concentrate on The Hundred and Rolling Back.

Progressing further

As you progress to more intense movements, you will drop some of the basic exercises you mastered at the beginning. This is because some of the beginners movements are built into the more advanced ones. So as you start doing The Seal, you will stop Rolling Back. Similarly, as you begin The Saw you will stop doing The Spine Twist. As before, keep on trying to do six or more exercises during the hour, picking an equal balance of strength and mobility movements from the chart as you progress. Always try to vary your selection and persist with the movements you find difficult. The better you become at doing Pilates exercises, the larger the choice of movement open to you becomes.

New Challenges Exercise Chart						
Page	Movement	Emphasis	Level 5	Level 6	Level 7	Level 8
54	THE PUSH-UP	Strength	o	o	o	o
56	SWIMMING	Strength	o	o	o	o
58	LEG PULL PRONE	Strength	o	o	o	o
60	ROLL-UP	Strength	o	o	o	o
62	ROLLING BACK	Mobility				
63	ONE LEG CIRCLE	Mobility	o	o	o	o
64	THE HUNDRED	Strength	o	o	o	o
66	THE SEAL	Mobility	o			
67	ONE LEG STRETCH	Strength	o	o		
68	THE SAW	Mobility	o	o	o	o
69	SHOULDER BRIDGE PREP	Mobility	o	o		
70	SIDE KICK	Strength	o	o	o	
71	SPINE STRETCH	Mobility	o	o	o	o
72	SPINE TWIST	Mobility	o	o	o	o
74	THE CRAB	Mobility	o	o	o	o
75	DOUBLE LEG STRETCH	Strength			o	o
76	ROCKER WITH OPEN LEGS	Mobility		o	o	o
77	SHOULDER BRIDGE	Strength			o	o
78	SIDE BEND	Strength	o	o	o	o
80	SIDE-KICK KNEELING	Strength				o
81	THE TEASER	Strength			o	o
82	JACK KNIFE	Strength				o
83	HIP TWIST	Strength			o	o
84	SCISSORS	Strength	o	o	o	o
85	THE ROCKER	Strength				o

If you have a known medical condition, are pregnant, or have any chronic joint problems, you should consult your doctor before starting any exercise program. It is not advisable to start Pilates after becoming pregnant unless you have already been training with the technique. A check-up is also advisable if you are aged over 40, if you are overweight or if have not been undertaking any physical exercise for some time. If you experience any chest pains or pain in your back or neck while doing any of the movements, then stop immediately. Drink plenty of fluids after you work out, especially in hot weather. Always wear comfortable clothes that will not restrict your movement.

Advanced Exercise Chart						
Page	Movement	Emphasis	Level 9	Level 10	Level 11	Level 12
54	PUSH-UP	Strength	o	o	o	o
56	SWIMMING	Strength	o	o	o	o
58	LEG PULL PRONE	Strength	o	o	o	o
60	ROLL-UP	Strength				
62	ROLLING BACK	Mobility				
63	ONE LEG CIRCLE	Mobility	o	o	o	o
64	THE HUNDRED	Strength	o	o	o	o
66	THE SEAL	Mobility				
67	ONE LEG STRETCH	Strength				
68	THE SAW	Mobility	o	o	o	o
69	SHOULDER BRIDGE PREP	Mobility				
70	SIDE KICK	Strength				
71	SPINE STRETCH	Mobility	o	o	o	o
72	SPINE TWIST	Mobility				
74	THE CRAB	Mobility				
75	DOUBLE LEG STRETCH	Strength	o	o	o	o
76	ROCKER WITH OPEN LEGS	Mobility	o	o	o	o
77	SHOULDER BRIDGE	Strength	o	o	o	o
78	SIDE BEND	Strength	o	o	o	o
80	SIDE-KICK KNEELING	Strength	o	o	o	o
81	THE TEASER	Strength	o	o	o	o
82	THE JACK KNIFE	Strength	o	o	o	o
83	HIP TWIST	Strength	o	o	o	o
84	SCISSORS	Strength	o	o	o	o
85	THE ROCKER	Strength	o	o	o	o
86	THE BOOMERANG	Mobility	o	o	o	o
87	NECK PULL	Strength	o	o	o	o
88	CONTROL BALANCE	Strength				o
89	LEG PULL SUPINE	Strength		o	o	o
90	THE CORKSCREW	Strength			o	o
91	ROLLOVER	Strength	o	o	o	o

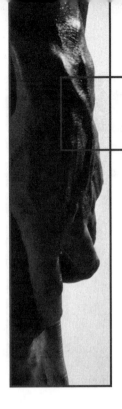

preventing pain

Pilates challenges us to examine how well our bodies are really functioning. Even the most healthy person may have niggling pains which indicate stresses and strains on the body. For others, the effects of ignoring the needs of our bodies is all too apparent. Pilates can help to build the body to prevent injury and help to keep us healthy through the development of good posture.

Most of us experience painful twinges in our bodies from time to time. These are little warning signals of trouble ahead. If we do not listen to our bodies, then the signals they give us can only become more insistent. Even those who are extremely fit, such as top athletes, can develop medical problems as a result of the body working in ways that are disharmonious. This is particularly true for golfers and tennis players who use one side of their bodies very differently from the other.

Muscle balance

Muscular stress is often hidden by groups of larger muscles that develop to protect weaker ones. This is the body's way of coping with a problem, but it is only ever short term. Pilates exercises will reveal the original source of the problem and address it directly. There are no short cuts to solving bad posture and back pain. For example, supporting devices, such as corsets, simply do the work that the muscles should be doing for themselves. We need to train our bodies to break their recourse to sloppy habits and learn new coping methods.

Pain and gain

These changes may at first feel uncomfortable but it is important to distinguish between this normal level of discomfort and the discomfort caused through the injury or problem itself. There is always a certain amount of discomfort that arises during training, especially when it comes to stretching muscles that you may not have used in some time. When stretching, it is best to think of discomfort along a scale of one to 10. Mild stretches rank one to four. From five on, you will be increasingly challenging yourself. A strong stretch may elicit some pain. Be careful not to push too far at the top end of the scale. If any pain is sudden or sharp you must stop immediately as this extreme should never be experienced. Only people who are very in tune with their bodies, such as dancers or sportspeople, work at the top end of the scale in order to push their performance levels to the limit. Pilates involves you finding out your own level of discomfort. Begin at the lower end of the scale, regardless of your overall level of fitness. I emphasize again that stretching exercises should be performed gradually. It is always better to build up slowly. Only in this way can you strike a balance between achievement and challenge. Never exercise when you are in chronic pain or when any of your muscles are inflamed. Remember to always seek medical advice for back problems as they can occur for a host of different reasons. Never self-diagnose.

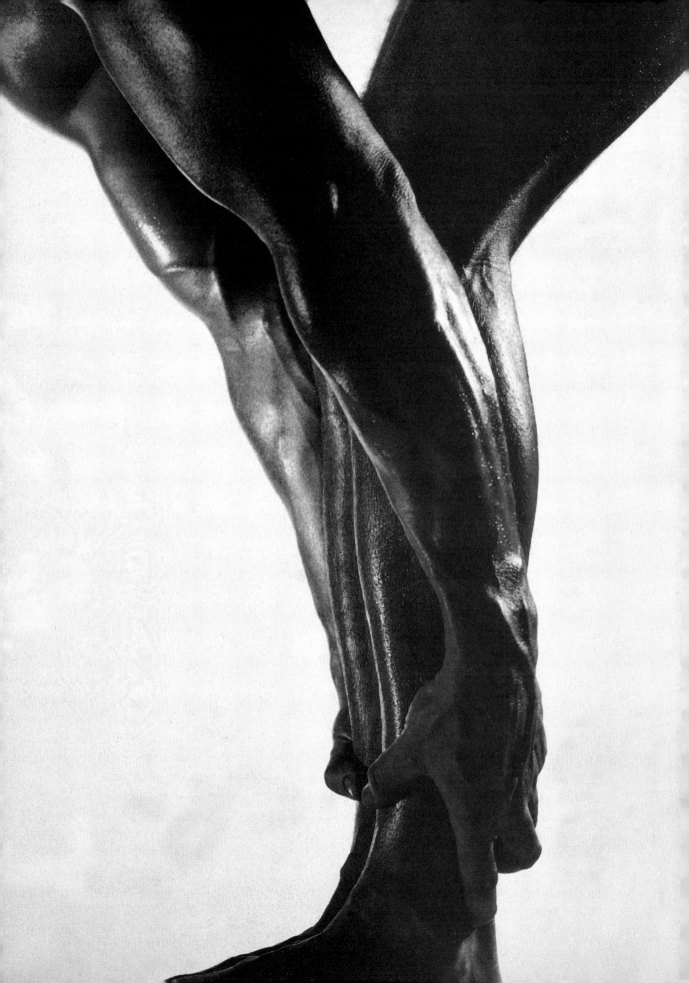

Your whole life

It is no good doing Pilates exercises for a few hours in the week if you spend the rest of your time slouched over a desk or slumped in front of the television. Pilates should make you think about the whole of your life and examine your everyday habits. Some of the suggestions set out here will complement your Pilates program and ensure that the philosophy of balance and control behind Pilates extends into the rest of your life.

Correct posture

Our postural habits develop from the moment we learn to walk. How we live our lives affects our posture, and all too often this means adopting bad posture. To rectify this, Pilates movements return us to the floor once again. This helps to reduce the strain of gravity so that we can build our strength. Correcting bad posture takes time and patience but the rewards of doing so are multifold. Your posture can directly affect your health. Even small stresses and strains can add up over a period of years to cause serious, permanent damage. Your back always reflects what you do to it.

Back pain

In the industrial world, the most common health problem among those under 65 is back pain. It has been estimated that our bodies are not designed to be static for more than twenty minutes at any given time, yet our modern lifestyles often entail long periods of sitting down, especially at work. One of

the things Joseph Pilates noticed about animals, especially cats, was the way they were constantly stretching their limbs and muscles. He believed that this was one of the reasons they remained so supple, nimble and poised. In the same way, humans need to keep moving and stretching.

Developing spine

Babies are born with spines that are shaped like commas, with just one curve. But as we mature, our spines adopt an S-shape, with a hollow at the base of our necks and another in the small of our backs. Try to keep these natural curves in the course of everyday life, even while sitting down. Review the way your everyday activites may be leading to bad posture. If you slouch, your spines forms an unhealthy C-shape. You can take precautionary measures by adopting better postural habits.

In the office

Modern sedentary working conditions mean that the average office worker may spend between 25 and 40 hours a week sitting down in a chair. Add this to the time we spend sitting to eat at a table, driving a car or slumped in front of the television and you get a sense of just how vital good posture is in our daily lives. A comfortable office chair cannot in itself compensate for poor posture. It is important to try to sit as erect as possible for as long as you can. Your feet should always be kept flat on the floor and it is best not to sit with your legs crossed for long periods. If you

are working at a computer, it is best to look slightly down at the screen. Your forearms should be in a horizontal position. Make sure the back of your seat supports your lumber curve; a small cushion can help support the lower back. This doesn't mean you must sit like a tin soldier all of the time. Make sure you get up from your desk as often as you can. Try not to spend more than twenty minutes working in the same position. Walk around the room to stretch your spine and improve your circulation. Try to organize your day so that it includes a series of natural breaks.

At home

While at home we undertake activities that can lead to back pain though bad posture. All working surfaces should be at the correct height. Kitchen sinks, for example, are often too low. This means we may need to stoop uncomfortably over them, causing stress in our lower backs. If yours is like this, try to raise the bowl to ensure there is no need to stoop over it. If there's a cupboard underneath the sink, rest one foot on the lower shelf. Keep changing your feet on the shelf to maintain the natural balance of your back.

Couch potatoes

When you are watching television, try to get up off the sofa for a stretch every half an hour. Throw away the remote control and get to your feet! Many sofas are built too low for the average adult. You should be able to sit with your back against the sofa back and your feet on the floor. If the seat is too deep, pack the space behind your lumbar curve with cushions.

Lying down

Your bed can dramatically effect the health of your back. Poor beds can in themselves lead to back pain. A good bed should support your spine so that it is level. Your natural S-shape should be maintained while lying on your back. Yet the mattress should also mould to the contours of your body. Your mattress should be neither too hard nor too soft. You can test this by seeing whether you can fit your hand underneath the curve of your back. It should fit easily between bed and back, neither being squeezed too tightly nor having too much room. The term "orthopedic" is used by mattress manufacturers to sell their products although this can be misleading. It is best to choose a comfortable mattress that is right for just you, rather than one that feels extra hard.

Driving

When we drive our cars we are often confined in a small space for hours on end. Most people experience back pain after lengthy car journeys. There are steps you can take to avoid this. Make sure your driving position is as comfortable as possible and that the controls are within easy reach. Do not hunch over the steering wheel or slouch in the seat but sit in an upright position. Make sure your mirrors are correctly adjusted so that you don't have to strain. It is best not to grip the wheel too tightly as this will tense your muscles and add to stress. You could also try pulling in your stomach muscles and breathing out, or try raising your shoulders towards your ears and pushing your shoulders down against the back of the seat.

Back exercises

CORE WORK

All these Pilates movements will strengthen your core, building strength in the muscles that support your spine

The hundred (p64)

Roll-up (p60)

Swimming (p56)

One leg stretch (p67)

The seal (p66)

Double leg stretch (p75)

Spine twist (p72)

OFFICE EXERCISE

• Pull in your chin, turn your head slowly to one side, without jerking it, before turning it to the opposite side. Repeat 3-4 times.
• Raise your shoulders up towards your ears then push them back and relax. Repeat 2-3 times.
• Tighten your abdominal muscles as you breathe out fully and count to five before releasing.
• When you are having a break from sitting down, stand with your feet apart and place your hands in the small of your back. Keeping your knees straight, push your hips forward and your shoulders back. This will release tension in the spine.

Avoiding back pain

PREVENTATIVE MEASURES

• Always aim to keep the normal S-shape curves of your spine in place for most of the day.
• Try to avoid hunching up your shoulders or slumping forward, causing your spine to form an unhealthy C-shape.
• Take frequent breaks to move around as much as you can. Try not to remain in a single fixed position for more than 30 minutes.
• Tuck in your abs as much as you can, especially when lifting something.
• To pick up heavy objects, bend your knees and keep your back straight; never bend over. Try to keep objects near to your body as you pick them up.

TO REDUCE PAIN

• Try to keep up your normal daily activities. Gentle exercise will strengthen your back muscles and improve flexibility. Avoid strenuous exercise such as aerobics.
• Try to avoid lifting heavy weights. Make several short trips to the shop rather than trying to carry heavy groceries all in one go.
• When sitting, both your feet should be resting on the ground. Do not cross your legs.
• If, after a few days, your pain persists, visit a qualified manipulative therapist such as an osteopath, chiropractor or physiotherapist.

vital elements

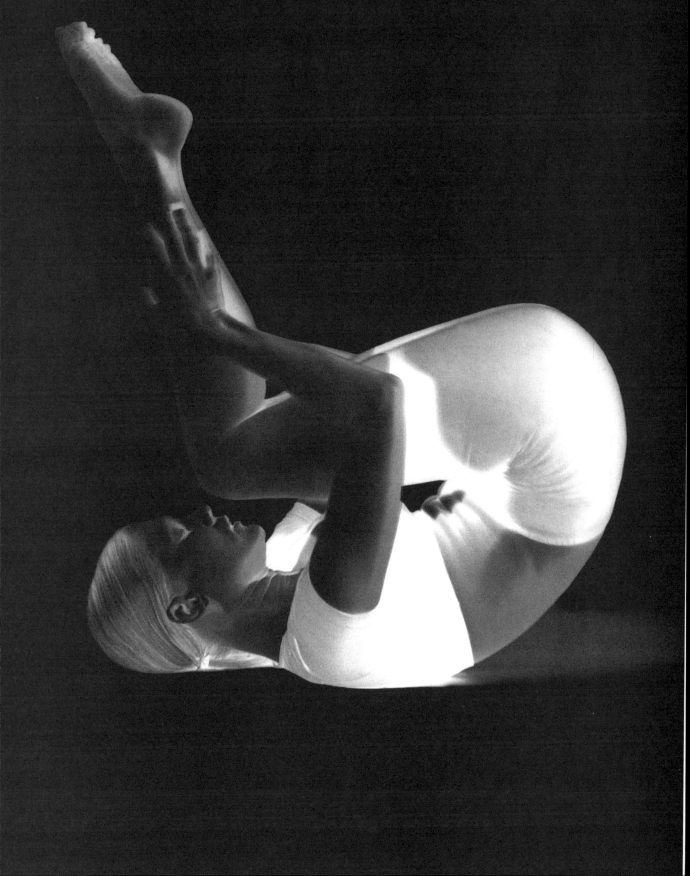

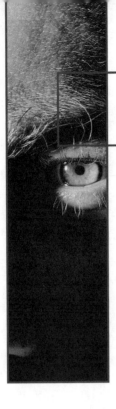

concentration

With many exercise classes and techniques you don't have to think about what you're doing, you just do it to get through it. But with Pilates, every movement is a conscious act controlled by the power of your mind.

"Always keep your mind wholly concentrated on the purpose of the exercises as you perform them." Joseph Pilates

Pilates is "the thinking way of moving" and requires a different kind of concentration than that typically used for other exercise forms. It may not be all that important to concentrate in this way during an aerobics class or when walking on a treadmill, but it is absolutely essential for Pilates.

Setting the mood

There are simple things you can do to improve concentration. Check that the space you plan to use for Pilates is free of distractions and that it is warm and comfortable. Make sure you will not be disturbed. Though Pilates is not a spiritual workout, you will find it very relaxing because concentrating hard on a single movement causes everything else that is going on in your life to fade away. If you want to use music in the background, make sure it isn't punctuated by a heavy beat. Do not make the

mistake I once made when I used a tape of nature sounds that featured screeching parrots and mating whales!

A clear mind

You'll soon find that the benefits of practicing concentration are well worth the effort—easier mental focus, clarity of thought and, most importantly, reduction of stress. All too often in our

whirlwind modern lives, visual clutter and noisy distractions make it hard for us to focus on the task at hand. Stress itself makes concentration more difficult (when you have too many things "on your mind") but persevere, as mental focus is an art that will improve with practice. Marshalling your powers of concentration will help you to feel more calm and in control.

Our inner voice

Controlling our thoughts, much like controlling our actions, is not as easy as it might first appear to be. When we are under pressure, our thoughts can become very erratic and spin off in random directions. If we are stressed, going to sleep can be especially difficult because we are unable to "switch off." Unwelcome thoughts pop into our heads despite our best efforts.

Effective concentration is a skill we acquire as children. By the time we are adults, we all have a little "inner voice" that controls our actions, for

example when we tell ourselves that we do like a particular exercise.

First attempts at unfamiliar movements may feel strange and awkward. It is very easy to fall into the trap of performing only the moves that you enjoy, when what you need most is to do the ones you do not like. Normally we speed up the difficult part of the movement to get it over with as soon as we can. Instead, we need to slow down. Only by concentrating hard on what you are doing can you properly control your actions.

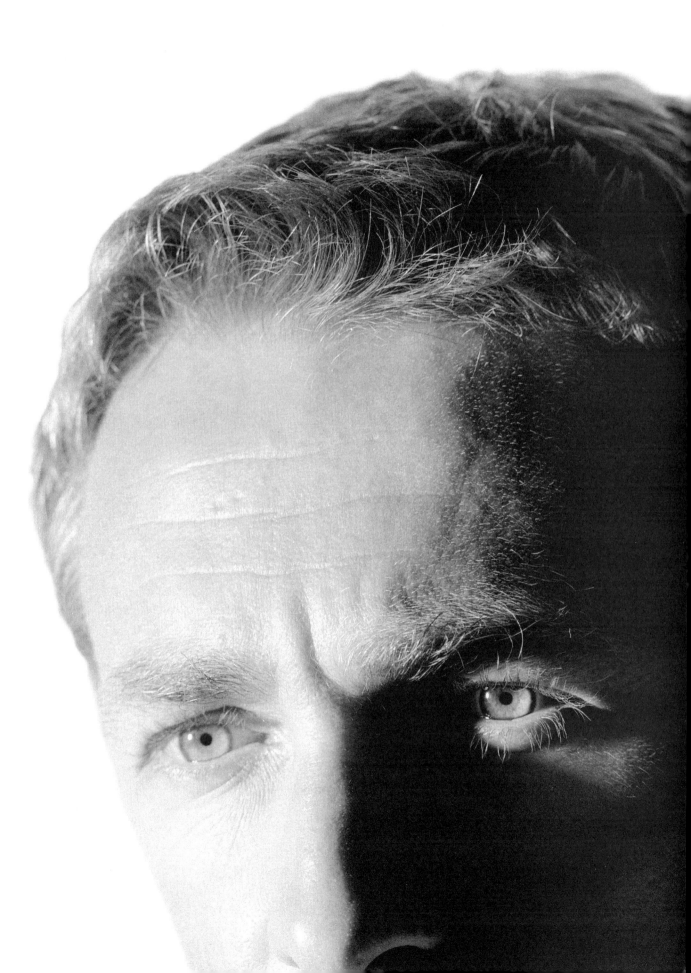

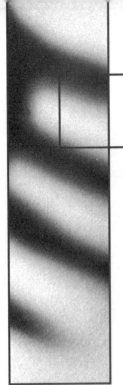

breathing

Pilates uses a controlled and continuous way of breathing that takes time to perfect, but results in a stronger and more energy-efficient body.

"Breathing is the first act of life. Our very life depends on it. Millions have never learned to master the art of correct breathing."

Joseph Pilates

Correct breathing takes time to master. Of all the vital elements, my students find this the most difficult to achieve and the last to fall into place. The main thing to remember is to breathe as frequently as you would naturally. If you find a movement is too slow for a single breath and you need to take another, take one.

Many Pilates instructors ask you to learn the breathing technique before learning the movements. My goal is the same, but my approach is different. I believe you can learn correct breathing while learning each of the movements.

The wrong way

Whatever you do, don't hold your breath. Most people hold their breath if they pick up something heavy, much as weightlifters would when picking up a barbell. This type of breathing is called the Valsalvic method and it results in a stressful increase in blood pressure. It wastes energy in parts of the body where it isn't required. Keep your breathing continuous.

Normal breathing

When you inhale normally, the lungs expand, the diaphragm drops and the stomach moves out. As you exhale, your diaphragm lifts and the stomach moves in. This is called "abdominal" breathing and is quite natural.

Pilates breathing

For Pilates you need to learn a new breathing technique. To strengthen the abdominals they must be contracted. This means abdominal breathing is not possible. Instead we use thoracic breathing (see below). Imagine you are wearing an invisible belt that is pulling your bellybutton towards your spine. Squeeze the stomach and breathe into the ribs.

Thoracic breathing

Try this breathing exercise. Sit comfortably on a chair or on the floor, with your legs crossed. Place your hands behind your back, with palms facing out and fingers touching your ribcage. Keeping your abdominals contracted, breathe in and feel your ribcage expand against your hands. Breathe in for two counts and out for two counts, repeating this several times. Now slow your breathing down to four counts for each in and out breath. Repeat this longer breath several times. Finally, try breathing in for eight counts and then out again for an equal eight counts. Aim to keep the abdominals contracted while breathing and breathe into your ribcage, rather than your stomach, so that the ribs expand outwards.

Or try this: place your right hand, palm down, on the lower front portion of your ribcage. Breathe into the one hand for eight counts, feeling your chest expand. Breathe out for eight. Repeat several times, change hands and repeat on the other side of your ribcage. Return to these exercises whenever the need arises.

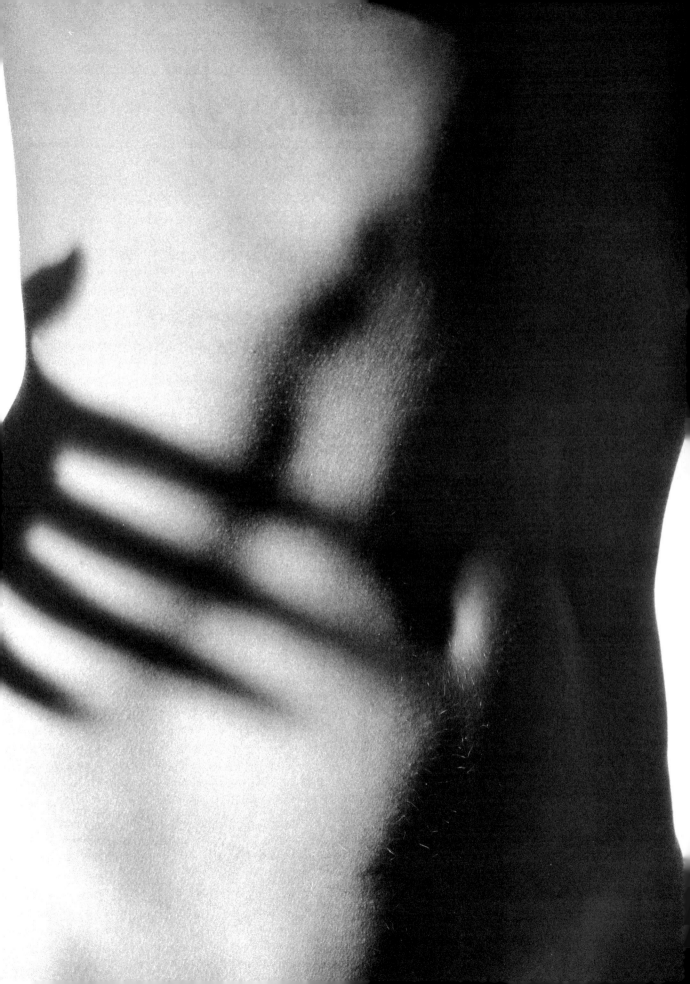

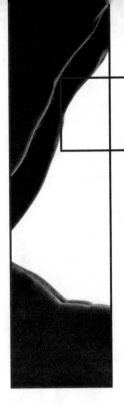

centering

The center of your body is the center of your power. The body should work in unison not as separate parts, with all movement stemming from your center.

"Pilates develops the body uniformly, corrects wrong postures, restores physical vitality, invigorates the mind and elevates the spirit." Joseph Pilates

Joseph Pilates believed that our abdominal muscles, now known as abs, function as the "powerhouse" for the whole of the body. Your abs are your center and they initiate every movement. To maintain a strong center you need an equal balance of strength, between the abs and the back.

Core essentials

When doing regular sit-ups we often think of moving first, then of pulling in our abs. We "crunch" these stomach muscles as we lift up. What we should actually be doing is contracting our muscles first and then moving our limbs. Ultimately every movement should be initiated by the contraction of your abs; whether you are lifting your arm or your leg, the movement starts here.

Think of a puppet. When you pull a string, its arm goes up. Your abdominals act as your "string." Strength flows outwards along

your limbs from this pivotal middle junction. Strong abs are the key to your body working as a unit and will help to strengthen all your other muscle groups.

Good foundations

Start each warm-up with the "Striking balance" exercise (below). You can also practice balancing correctly the next time you are waiting in a supermarket

queue. Your feet support your body most effectively when they lie directly under your hips so that you can balance evenly on the ball of each foot, the outside edge of the foot and the center of your heel. Women who usually wear high heels tend to lean backwards to compensate for the shoes' forward pitch. Ideally you should not push too far forward from your heels or back from your toes.

Striking balance

Stand with your bare feet shoulder-width apart. Lift your toes as high as you can. Imagine a triangle between your big toe, little toe and heel. Place this imaginary triangle evenly on the ground, letting your toes drop and spread out. Open your shoulders, lengthen your spine and imagine a string, attached to the top of your head, pulling you up to the ceiling.

Pull in your abs and breathe out as you push up onto the balls of your feet. Stretch up, as tall as possible. Then slowly lower your heels. Make sure your toes stay relaxed and don't

crunch up. When your heels just touch the ground, keep your body weight in that position. Your body is now centered.

It might feel like you are leaning forward. This is because we are so accustomed to putting our weight on our heels. If you could look sideways in a mirror you should be able to draw a straight line vertically from your shoulders to your hips to the middle of your feet. To maintain this posture you have to keep your abdominals contracted, which makes the body work harder.

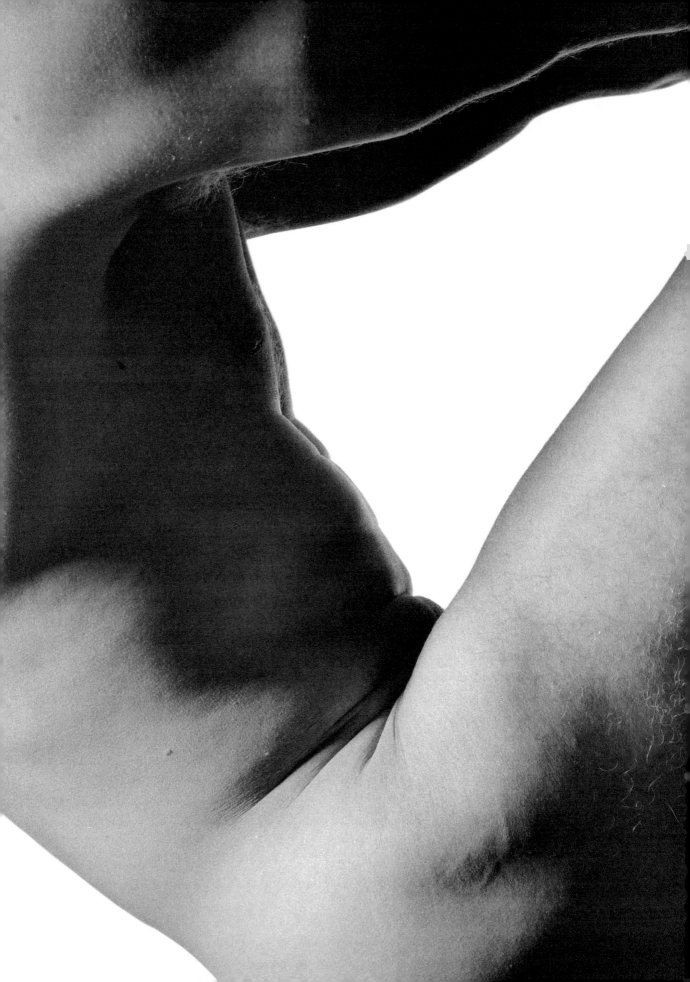

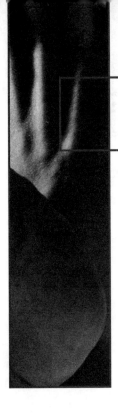

control

We start learning control when we take our first shaky steps as a child. Far from constricting us, good control frees our potential and teaches us how to take charge of our own bodies and fulfil our physical capabilities.

"Good posture can be successfully acquired only when the entire mechanism of the body is under perfect control." Joseph Pilates

Imagine a child walking for the first time, staggering forward with arms stretched out. At this early age, on learning to walk, we are training our bodies to resist the pull of gravity. We begin developing strength and control and, as we get stronger, we walk with more skill. Over time our postural habits develop, but often not as they should. Through Pilates, we can go back a step and re-learn the art of control.

Go slow

All Pilates movements are slow and controlled. They should be done at the same constant speed throughout. None of the actions are jerky or frenetic as this puts your body at risk of injury. Slower movements are much harder to control and are, therefore, more exacting and ultimately more effective. Practicing Pilates will show you how little you previously thought about your movements.

Perfect visuals

Imagine a man doing a bicep curl. His muscles are tense as he lifts the dumbbell, and then, quite often, the arm just relaxes and swings back down. If the down movement is uncontrolled, he only gains partial benefit from the workout. He also risks injury. In Pilates, control should be used at every point of the movement.

Think now of a gymnast standing on a narrow balance beam. She performs a forward roll and ends once again in a standing position. Her control and precision keep her from falling off, helping her to maintain a constant speed as she rolls. Visualizing images can help you to understand control and maximize your workout. Use this image and work towards the same quality of movement in your Pilates. Try the "Resist me" exercise (below) to see how effective visualization can be.

Resist me

Find a partner. Stand up, holding a towel in your right hand. Have your partner sit down at your feet and hold the other end of the towel with both hands. Pull your fist, with the towel, towards your shoulder in a bicep curl. Let your partner create resistance so that there is equal tension as you move your arm up and down.

Think about a resistance scale from one to 10. One is when your partner exerts no resistance with the towel.

10 is when your partner pulls so hard that you can't move at all. Aim for a resistance level of five in both directions. Breathe out as you curl the arm up and breathe in as you uncurl the muscle. Repeat 10 times and change arms.

Next, drop the towel but imagine you are still holding it and repeat the bicep curl. Do you feel the resistance that you had when you were holding the towel? This visualization technique will aid controlled action.

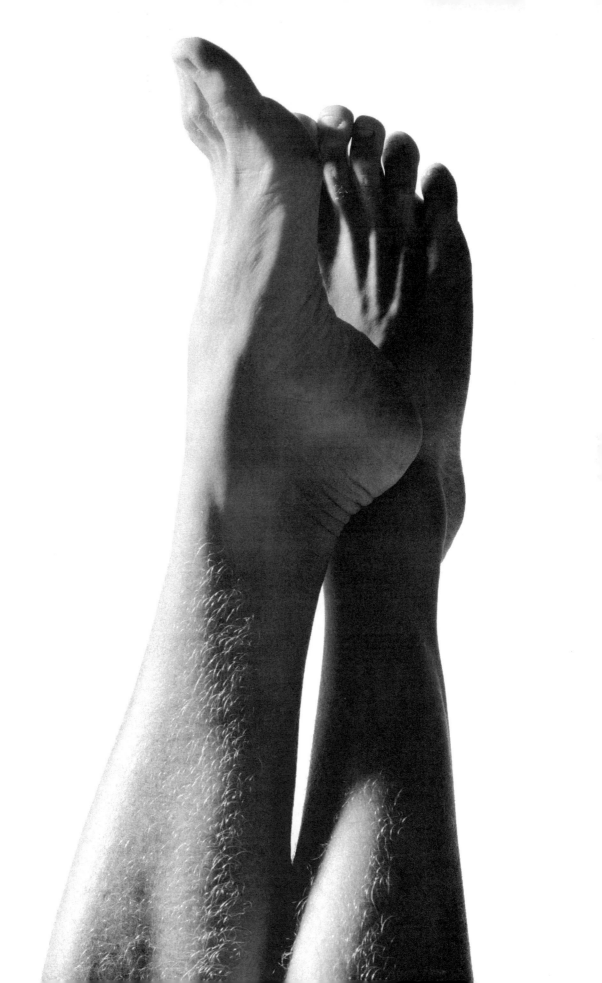

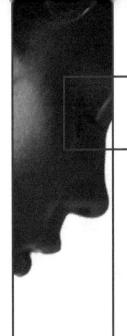

precision

Everybody has their own natural geometry. Pilates can help us to move with more precision and discover for ourselves the dimensions of natural grace.

"The benefits of Pilates depends solely on your performing the exercises exactly according to the instructions."

Joseph Pilates

All Pilates movements are exact, and involve precise actions and precise breathing. When you think of precision and movement, you might think of synchronized swimmers or the exacting choreography that dancers can achieve. Remember that Joseph Pilates trained as both a boxer and an acrobatic circus performer. This gave him an appreciation of precision skills and an acute awareness of space and time.

Catching the moment

The most dramatic example of precision I have ever witnessed was the Cirque de Soleil show called "O" in Las Vegas. The piece combines the precise acrobatic skills of the performers with advanced stage technology. Accuracy was vital in the performance, not just for effect but also for the safety of the performers. To my joy, as I looked through the program of this incredible event, I saw that two full-time Pilates instructors were listed as staff members. This level of physical activity requires extreme concentration, but we can all practice precision to some degree through Pilates.

Perfect reach

Bring to mind the image of the spread-eagled figure drawn by Leonardo da Vinci. The artist has drawn a circle around the figure as he stretches out to his fullest extent. These lines of geometry are a useful visualization of the space around us.

Usually we are unaware of the space we occupy and how our movements take place within it. Because Pilates demands that you not only move correctly, but breathe correctly, you will become more aware as to how your personal space is created through concentration and the use of precision. It is through precision

Spot on

My version of the popular game *Pin the Tail on the Donkey* requires no donkey and no pin. Just stand up and find a spot on the door in front of you. Slowly reach out with your right arm and touch the spot. As you bring your right arm back, begin stretching your left arm out to touch the same point. Repeat for 30 seconds, keeping the alternate movement of the two arms continuous. Do not stop and make sure the elbows do not lock.

Now turn around and imagine that same point but in an imaginary space in front of you. Focus on that spot and again reach for it with your right hand, alternating with your left hand, but without the help of the visual cue. Keep going for at least another 30 seconds, always aiming for the same point in space. You have just practiced precision.

that we can attain grace of movement. Imagine the arm of a ballet dancer arching like the tip of a compass; we are all capable of making pin points in space.

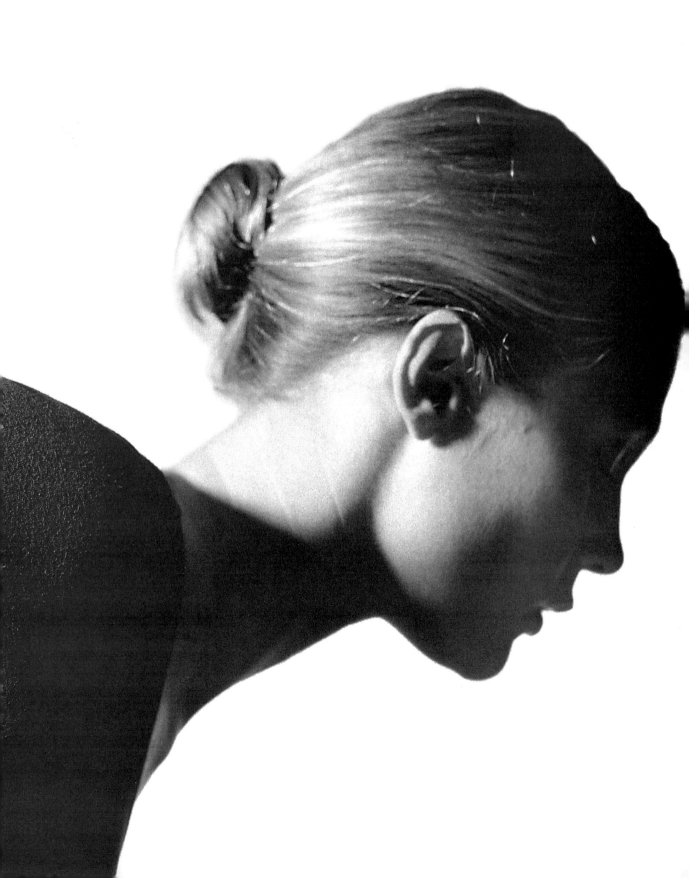

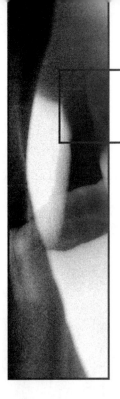

movement

Think slow, controlled and continuous movements. Imagine a wheel turning slowly, never speeding up or slowing down, and never pausing.

"Designed to give you suppleness, grace and skill that will be unmistakably reflected in the way you walk, the way you play, and in the way you work." Joseph Pilates

When I explain to new students the type of movement required for Pilates exercises, I always compare it to tai chi. It is slow, graceful and controlled. As with tai chi, all Pilates movements are continuous: they have no beginning and no end. Nothing is sharp, strained or forced.

No sweat

With many exercise techniques the focus is on repetition and you stop after each one. Pilates movements are different in that you don't pause until you have completed the required number of repetitions. Each movement is a long, continuous cycle as this requires greater skill to control. If you need to be convinced that slow, controlled movements are more difficult, try the "Slower is harder" challenge (right). The truth is that there is no need for you to work up a sweat or exercise at speed for it to be effective!

Full range

This type of movement can be applied to other forms of exercise with much success: try using resistance machines or free weights in the gym with slow, steady and even movements. You will be able to feel the difference and it will prove more effective (you may have to use a lighter weight). It is also vitally important to ensure that you are using your full range of movement. Check that you are working equally hard, with the same intensity and resistance throughout. As much effort should be used to extend a muscle (eccentric movement) as to contract it (concentric movement). By working in this way, you will begin to develop strength and flexibility in equal measure, giving your muscles (and your body) a long, lean look.

Slower is harder

Begin by doing five regular push-ups (press-ups), either with your legs fully extended in the full push-up position, or with your knees on the floor (the three-quarter position). Do these first five at your normal pace.

Now do another five, but count two slow counts down and two slow counts up. Breathe in as you go down and out as you come up. Rest. Now repeat, but to a count of four in each direction. Rest. Finally, try a last five push-ups, to a count of six on the way down and another six on the way up, without pausing at the top or at the bottom, making all five push-ups one long, continuous and steady movement. It was harder than you thought, wasn't it?

At this latter point you are working at the same intensity that you should be working at while doing the Pilates exercises. It is all about quality and range of movement, with the contraction of the muscles (the downward movement in this case) and the flexion (the pushing up movement) requiring equal effort.

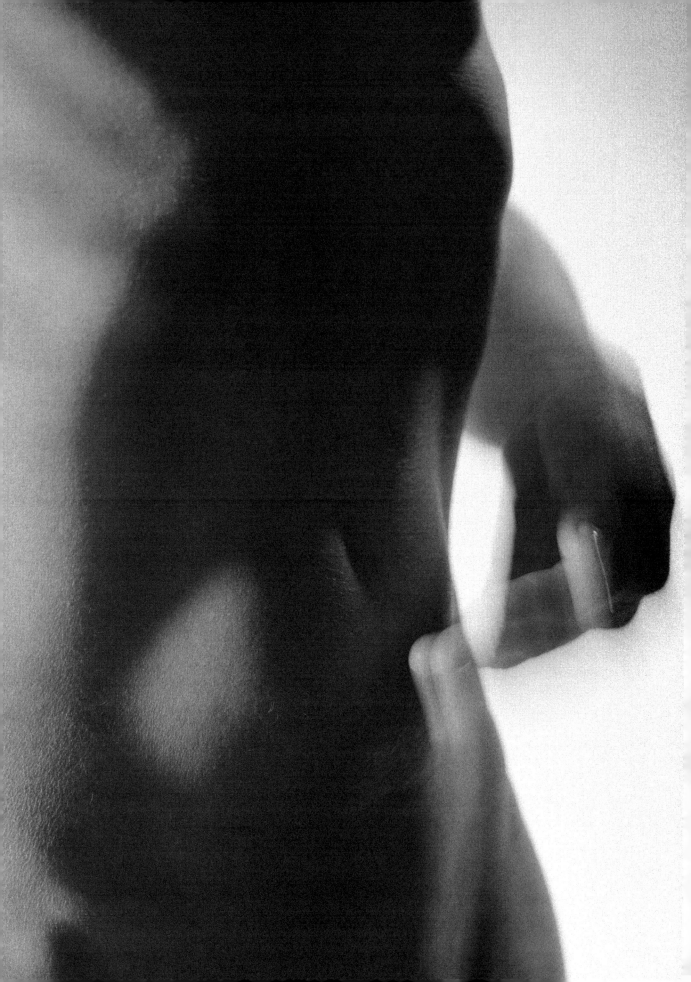

isolation

The Pilates technique is an excellent way of educating yourself and understanding, through movement, how your body works, in part and as a whole. Harmony comes from the integration of isolated parts.

"Each muscle may cooperatively and loyally aid in the uniform development of all our muscles." Joseph Pilates

For many years exercise teachers have talked about isolating different muscles. Yet it is only theoretically possible to see them in isolation; in practice, all our muscles work together in groups. Again, in regular exercise classes, we have also talked about "spot reducing" certain areas to achieve a desired look. But in doing this we develop one muscle at the expense of another. Consequently, the whole balance of the body is thrown. This "lopsided" approach is altogether at odds with the logic of the Pilates method.

Muscle balance

When we talk about isolation in Pilates we are simply making sure that we identify all our muscles for ourselves, especially the weaker ones. Pilates exercises ensure we develop the neglected areas of the body that work alongside opposing, stronger muscles. For example, if you are a golfer, you know that when you play you only swing in one direction. Over a period of time your body will become over-trained in this direction. Although we don't all play golf, we do all harbor muscle imbalances to some degree. It is not uncommon to discover these over- or under-trained areas through Pilates.

Weak links

Try to be aware of any imbalance in muscle strength or flexibility as you perform the movements and work towards the weaker of the two sets of muscles, so that balance is eventually regained. Otherwise, as you get stronger you will remain proportionally imbalanced. Try the "Touch and visualize" exercise to better understand how muscles work. Learn to identify the location of, say, your tricep without actually having to touch it. Visualization techniques will help you to

Touch and visualize

Sit down on a chair with a dumbbell, or bag of sugar or bottle of water to use as a weight. Sitting upright, hold the weight above your head in the right hand, with your right arm stretched straight towards the ceiling. Bring the left hand up to touch the back of your upper right arm with the tips of your fingers, keeping your right elbow close to your head. Lower the weight slightly behind your head and lift it back again to the ceiling. With the fingers of your left hand feel the tricep muscle at the back of the arm contracting and extending. Repeat 10–20 times. Now shift the weight to the other hand and repeat.

Finally, repeat the movement without the weight and without touching the triceps. Try and visualize the muscle working, from what you have just experienced.

connect mentally with the muscle. Over time you will be able to feel and identify various muscles working in combination as you perform the movements.

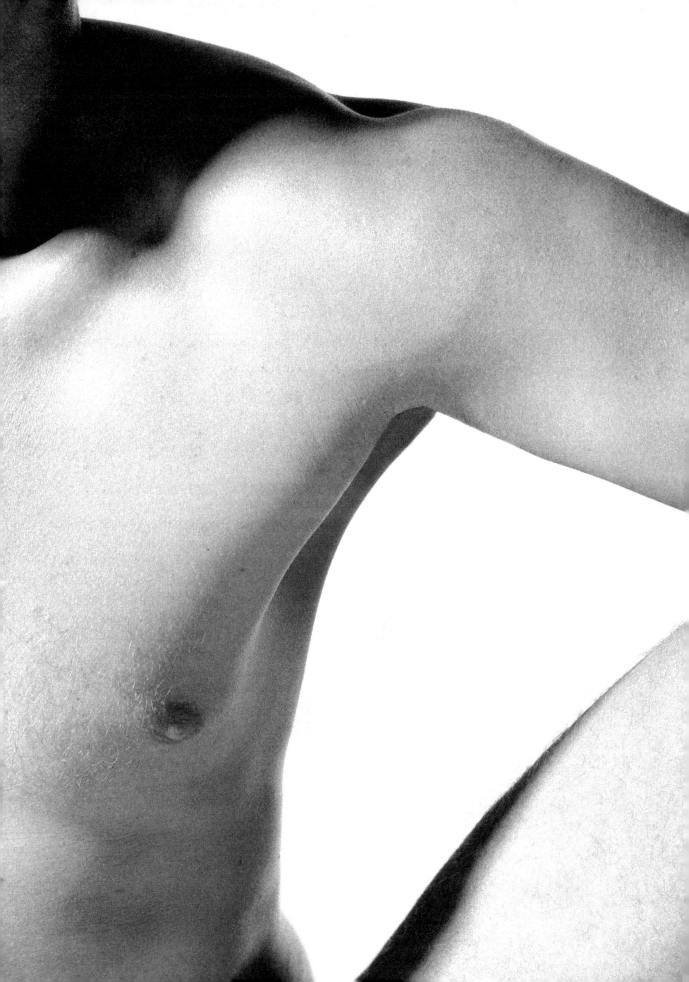

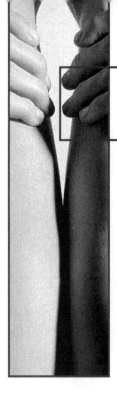

routine

Pilates is not an "instead of" but an "as well as"—it does not replace your current exercise program, but rather complements and enhances it by improving the way your muscles work together. But you must practice!

"Make up your mind that you will perform your Pilates movements 10 minutes [each day] without fail." Joseph Pilates

The development of a routine will help you get the best from Pilates. It does not promise quick-fix solutions but it does achieve real results by offering a gentle overhaul of your daily habits.

Making time

I often hear people say "I don't have time to exercise." But I have found that the easiest way to help my clients develop a routine is for them to treat Pilates as an important business appointment. They schedule it into their diaries as they would any other meeting. Devoting thirty minutes every day to the maintenance of your body is scant attention, especially when you stop to consider what you ask your body to do for you. We often treat our cars with more care than we do our bodies. Yet there is no question of trading in your body for a new model! Sticking to a routine is a way of taking yourself and your body seriously.

Regular slots

People often ask me, "How often should I do it?" and there is no easy answer. Like anything, the more you do it, the more quickly you will see results. Look at your goals and other commitments and decide how much time you can you can really dedicate to Pilates. Then be patient as you develop a regular routine. Bear in mind that Pilates in itself is not a replacement for cardiovascular activities and should always be combined with a balanced workout program. Gradually you will feel the muscles around your hips and waist tighten and tone as your body shape begins to change. Doing Pilates two or three times a week will also add to the effectiveness of other exercise programs as it promotes strength, flexibility and balance.

Practice makes perfect

Many of my clients want to know when their bodies will begin to look different. I always say, "If you've done the striking balance exercise, you will already look different. But maintaining good posture takes time."

We want instant results but, as with everything else, progress takes time and practice. Think of it as being like learning to drive. We need to develop new skills, and the more lessons and experience we have, the better drivers we become. It is exactly the same with your body and Pilates.

When you practice this technique your muscles will become leaner through regular stretching. Pilates not only changes body shape but will also increase your body strength.

Although we often look for cosmetic results, Pilates places just as much importance on the fundamental realignment of our bodies that will make them more flexible and pain-free. This process is not a magical one but simply the logical result of training your body to behave in new and more balanced ways.

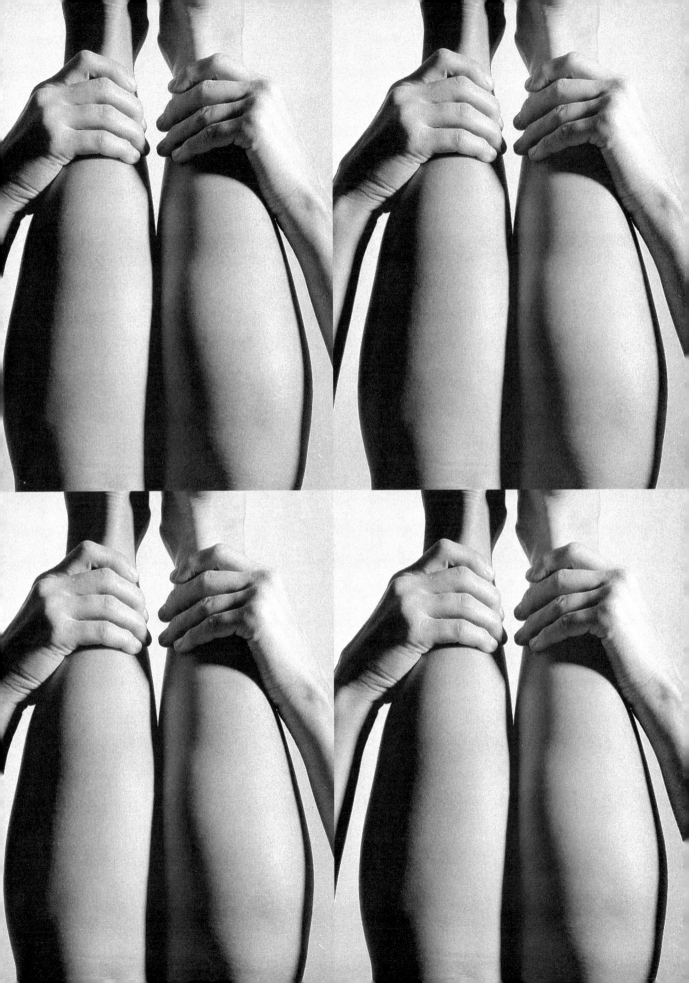

movements

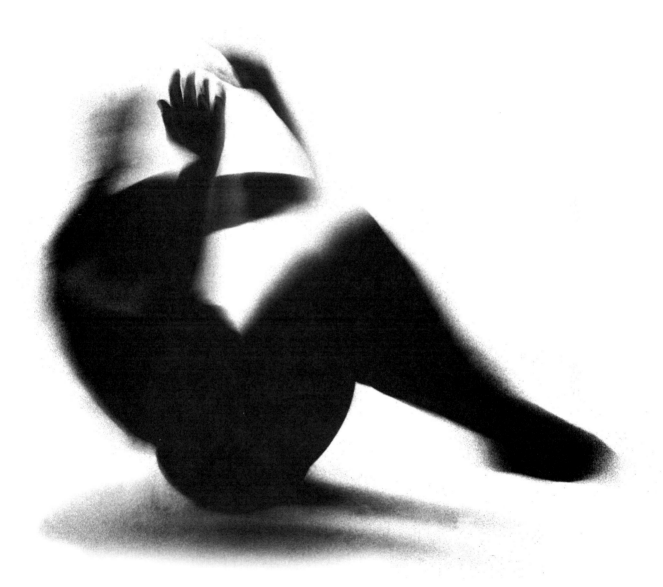

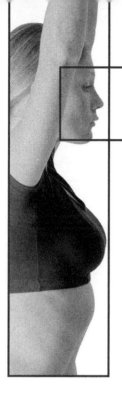

warm-ups

The warm-up is an essential part of your regular program and should precede every session of Pilates. Warming up prepares your body for the movements ahead by improving the blood flow from your heart to your muscles. Use this time to concentrate on your body. Shut out the events of the day and focus on your posture and movements.

swinging

This movement will warm up your spine and back muscles. Be gentle with yourself and do not force the body. Move slowly and with control, as if you were moving through water.

emphasis	mobility
visual cue	low bow
repeat	20 times

1 With your feet apart and knees relaxed, stretch your arms up to the ceiling, but not past your head. Pull in your abs.

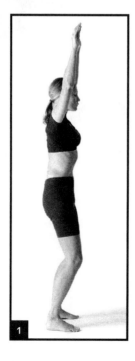

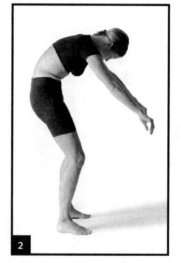

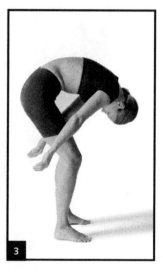

2 Breathe out and let your arms fall forward past your head. As they swing, allow your knees to bend and your back to curve. Relax your head and shoulders and pay attention to your spine as it gently relaxes, curling over. Keep your abs tight and the movement gentle.

3 After reaching the curled position, breathe in and roll slowly back up to the standing position. Each time you repeat the movement, try to stretch a little further toward the ceiling. Imagine a string is attached to the top of your head, pulling your entire body upwards.

round back

This movement will release your back.

■ CAUTION

Begin with small movements and gradually allow them to build in size. Do not force the movement and always keep your abs tucked in.

emphasis	mobility
visual cue	cat stretch
repeat	10 times

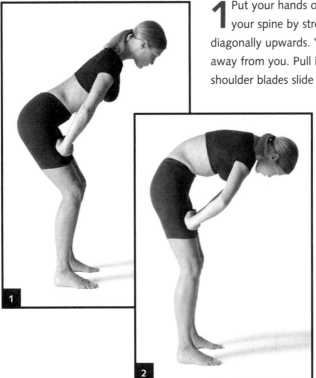

1 Put your hands on your thighs and lengthen your spine by stretching your head and neck diagonally upwards. Your tail bone should curl away from you. Pull in your abs and let your shoulder blades slide down your back.

2 Breathe out and gently round your back. Imagine a string attached to your waistband, pulling you up and backwards. Repeat the warm-up without stopping; keep working in a single continuous movement. Breathe in as you return to the starting position and be sure to avoid hollowing your back in the opposite direction.

chest stretch

This movement warms up the chest muscles. Do not reach the same point each time but try and spread your arms further. Visualize that you are creating space in the joints.

emphasis	mobility
visual cue	cutting a "V" shape
repeat	10 times

1 Stand tall with your feet apart, knees soft and your arms stretched out with palms up in front of you. Breathe in.

2 Breathe out and stretch your arms up and to the sides. Keep your spine long by pulling that invisible string to the ceiling. As you open your arms check that you are contracting your abs. Do not let your back arch. Keep the movement slow and the speed constant.

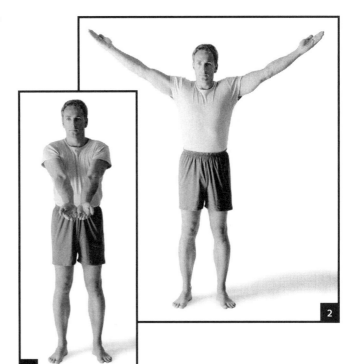

one arm circles

This movement opens up the shoulder joints.

❚ CAUTION

Do not lock your elbows and always work within your limits. If you find that you are able to make bigger circles on one side than the other, work on the weaker side in order to achieve balance in the body.

emphasis	mobility
visual cue	drawing circles
repeat	10 times each side

1 Stand tall with your feet apart, knees soft. Reach up from the top of your head to the ceiling to check that your back is correctly aligned. Keeping your right arm by your side, pressed lightly against the leg, breathe in and lift your left arm in front of you and slightly to the side.

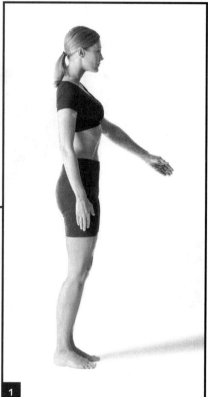

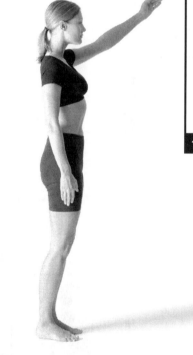

2 Keeping the ribcage still, start to draw a circle with the arm as you breathe out. If the ribcage moves, you are swinging too far—move the arm further away from the body to the side and draw a smaller circle. Imagine you are drawing on the wall to the side of you with the tips of your fingers.

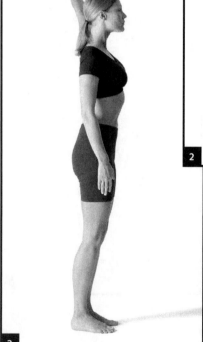

3 Complete the circle, trying at all times to keep a slow, consistent speed. Imagine a wheel turning, with continuous motion and no sudden jolts. When you have completed 10 circles on one arm, change arms and repeat.

double arm circles

emphasis	mobility
visual cue	arm hoops
repeat	10 times

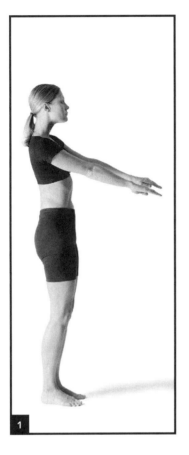

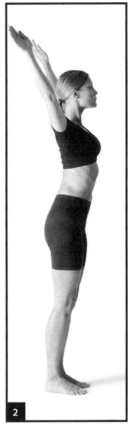

1 Stand tall with your feet apart, knees soft. Start with your arms slightly in front of you. Keep your abs pulled in and check that your back is in alignment.

2 Breathe out slowly and circle both arms back. Try to keep your hands together as you reach to the ceiling. Check your back does not arch by keeping your abs pulled in as tightly as possible.

3 Keep the speed of your movement constant and try to increase the size of the circle. When you reach 10, repeat in the opposite direction.

toy soldier

emphasis	mobility
visual cue	air paddle
repeat	10 times

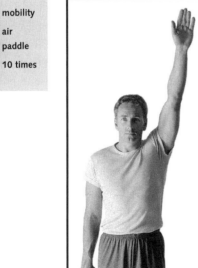

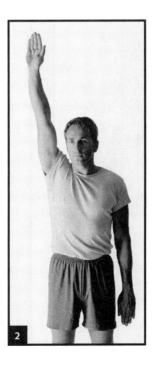

1 Stand tall with your feet apart and knees soft. Breathe in. Reach your left arm to the ceiling and your right arm to the ground.

2 Breath out as you bring the lifted arm forwards and down, swapping to lift the lower arm up to the ceiling. Keep your torso still and stretch the top of your head to the ceiling. Keep the speed slow and the action smooth. Repeat 10 times.

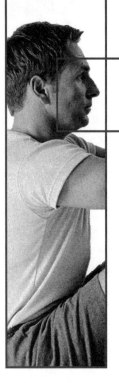

the essentials

The following movements are the building blocks of the Pilates technique. As always, start with the easier alternatives and work your way up to the pure version of the movement. Take time to work through each exercise. Listen to your body—you should never struggle to complete any of the movements. It is always best to develop strength slowly but surely.

push-up

Think of this as one long and continuous slow movement. The speed is very important. Try slowing down the movement each time in order to challenge yourself.

█ CAUTION

Find out where you need to put your hands in order to maintain control.

emphasis	strength
visual cue	snail on wall
repeat	10 times

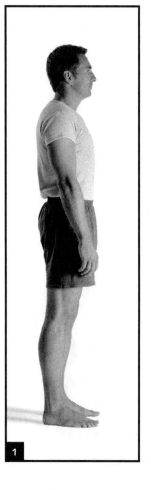

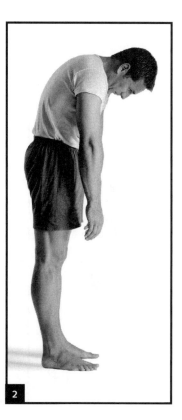

1 Stand tall with your feet apart, knees soft. Breathe in and contract your abs as you prepare to start slowly rolling your head and trunk down.

2 If you know you have tightness in a certain area of your back, slow down as you pass through that area. Keep your abs pulled in. Imagine you are leaning against a wall so that your butt does not push back. It should feel as though you are folding in on yourself.

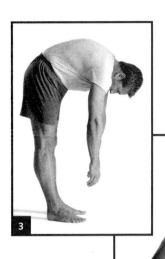

3 As you roll down, try to go as far as you can without forcing the stretch. If you feel any uncomfortable strain on your back, bend your knees slightly to release stress in your back.

4 If you cannot touch the floor at the furthest point of your roll down, bend your knees and lean forwards. On contact, breathe out and walk your hands forward on the floor.

5 Keep the movement slow, smooth, and gentle, as if you are trying to be silent.

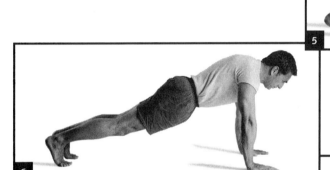

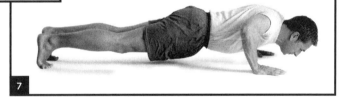

6 Stop walking when your hands are at shoulder level. Stretch longer by sliding your shoulders down your back, keeping your body straight.

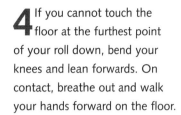

7 Breathe in and bend your arms to lower your chest toward the floor. Breathe out as you push back up and then walk your arms back and uncurl, reversing steps 6 to 1.

push-up alternative

If this movement at first proves too challenging, and you cannot complete a full stretch push-up, then drop to your knees for positions 6 and 7. The closer your hands are to the legs the easier the push-up will be. As your strength builds, work up to the straight leg version.

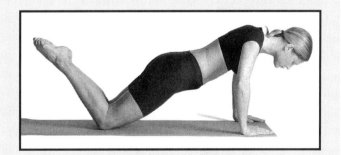

swimming

Imagine you have a piece of paper passing under your abs. Try not to touch it with your stomach. Find how high you can move without letting your abs touch the mat.

■CAUTION

Keep elbows soft. There should be no pressure in the lower back. Do not hunch the shoulders.

emphasis	strength
visual cue	diagonal switch
repeat	10 times

56

THE ESSENTIALS

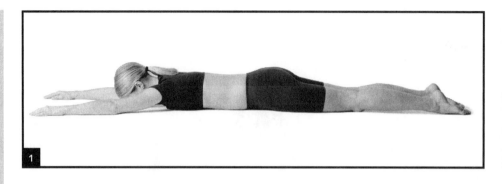

1 Lying face down, stretch the top of your head forward and slide your shoulders down your back. Stretch your legs behind you keeping them hip-width apart and contract your abs to lift your navel off the floor. This is the position you must try to maintain throughout the movement.

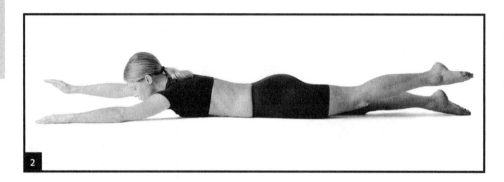

2 Breathe out as you lift your left leg and right arm up and away from you. Lift your limbs as high as you can without touching the mat with your navel. Feel your muscles lengthening along the floor before you lift. Do not struggle to lift too high as the lengthening is more important.

3 Breathing in, lower the limbs to change to the other side. Your little finger and little toe should be on the same diagonal line in space. Keep the movement slow and controlled. The speed of the movement should stay the same on both the lifting and the lowering of your limbs.

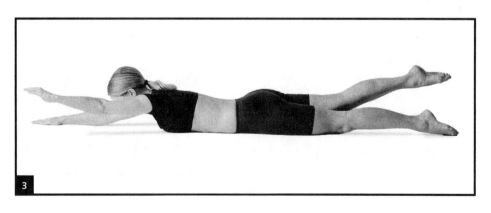

swimming alternatives

Try these easier alternatives if you feel any stress or pain in the lower back. Instead of lifting your abs keep them on the ground. This will limit the scope of the movement. Focus on your center and not your legs as you move. Work toward lifting your abs by visualizing that the floor is hot and that you do not want to burn your navel.

The aim is always to maintain a neutral spine in a face-down position (see page 73 for a description of the neutral spine). As this movement is hard to achieve for some, you may find yourself crossing the line from control to struggle. Avoid this by taking your time. Push your legs and arms into the floor before you try to lift them.

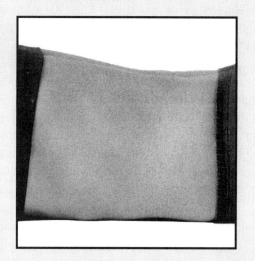

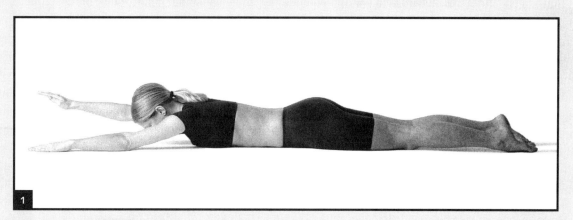

1 Isolate the upper body by keeping both legs down. Breathe out as you lift your head and right arm up and away from the floor. Breathe in as you lower your arm and swap to the left. Your goal is to keep your navel off the mat.

2 Isolate the lower body by putting your head on your arms in front of you. Slide your shoulders down your back. Breathe out as you lift the right leg away from you. Tighten the stomach and lift off the floor. Lower the right leg and change to the left.

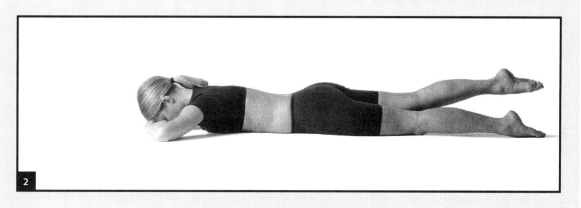

leg pull prone

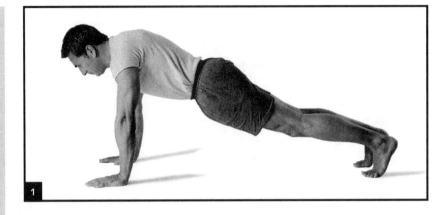

1 Start in a push-up position with your back in a straight line and your abs tucked in to protect your back. Be sure not to let your butt lift higher than your shoulders. Keep your shoulders pulled down and held in place; do not lock your elbows. Breathe in.

2 Breathe out as you raise your right leg, not letting your hips move. Initiate the lift by contracting your abs. Pretend you are a puppet: when you pull the string of the puppet the leg lifts. Your string is your abs being tightened.

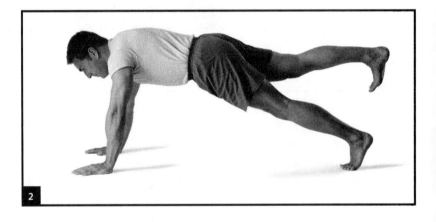

3 Breathe in as you lower the leg and breathe out as you change to lift up the other leg. Your goal should be to make sure that your hips do not move. Keep your back straight. Check that your shoulders are pulled down your back and that your neck is stretched. Legs should be lifted and lowered slowly and continuously, with no change in speed.

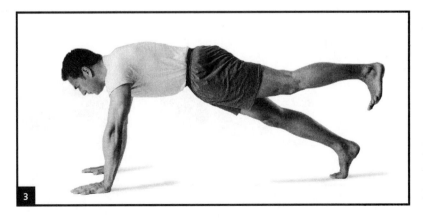

THE ESSENTIALS

leg pull prone alternatives

ALTERNATIVE 1

Rest your forearms on the ground, placing them as wide apart as your shoulders. Because you are now nearer the floor, the pull of gravity is less and you will find the leg moves easier to control. Try to keep your balance and keep the motion smooth.

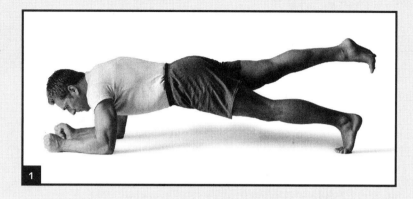

ALTERNATIVE 2

1 If the leg lifting proves too difficult at first, try practicing your balance by holding this position. Place your forearms firmly on the floor and curl your toes. Toes and hands should be aligned.

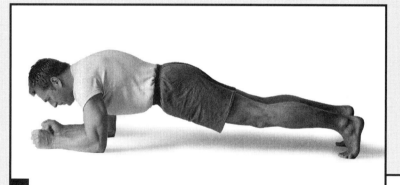

2 For a less intense version, place your knees on the ground also. Remember to keep your abs tucked in and hold your bottom down in line with your shoulders.

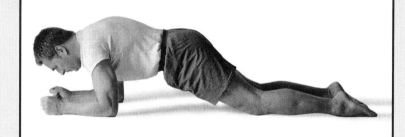

3 To reduce the intensity even further, lower the hips down. You should be resting the weight of your lower body on both of your feet. Tuck in your abs and feel your weight shifting as you push down on your arms.

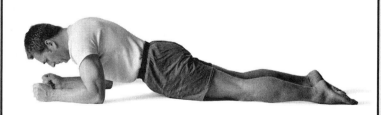

roll-up

This movement is intended to develop your abdominal strength.

⚠ CAUTION

If it proves too difficult to roll up off the floor then you will need to focus more on the mobility of your back. Do not attempt to force this move or struggle to complete it.

emphasis	strength
visual cue	rising sun
repeat	10 times

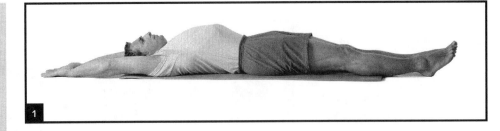

1 Lie on the floor on your back with your legs straight and stretch your arms above your head. Check that your shoulders are pulled down your back.

2 Slowly lift your arms to the ceiling as you breathe in. Try to keep a neutral spine (see page 73 for description of this) as your arms lift up.

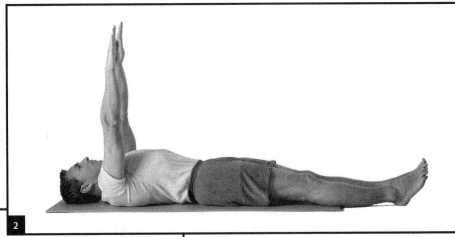

3 Breathe out and slowly roll forward, peeling your spine off the mat. Keep your head in alignment and let your eyes lead the way. Keep your trunk taught and do not crunch the body.

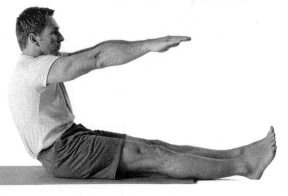

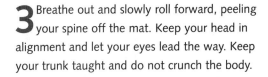

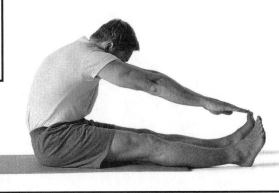

4 Stretch out over your legs as you breathe in, then slowly roll back down to the floor as you breathe out. Do not pause but continue to roll up again, each time trying to reach a little further toward your toes.

roll-up alternatives

This variation allows you to start at a lower level as your strength builds and the flexibility in your back improves. You will be able to stretch a little further every time you return to this movement. Remember to keep your feet firmly set on the floor at all times.

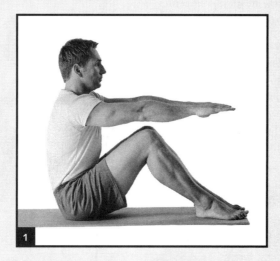

1 Start from a seated position with your arms stretched out in front of you. Sit tall as if you have a hook at the top of the head which is pulling you up toward the ceiling. Slide your shoulders down your back and position your legs with knees bent, at a comfortable distance from your body. You should be able to sit without hunching your shoulders.

2 Breathe in and roll back to the point where you feel you can still keep control of the movement. This will be determined by the flexibility of your back and the strength in your center. Breathe out on your return to the seated position. Do not stop at this point. Keep moving and complete 10 movements. As you become more flexible you will be able to lean further back.

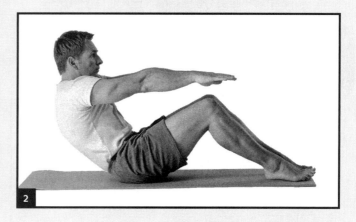

listen to your body

Our bodies are never the same day-to-day and so you should expect your capabilities to vary. Working out on a Friday, after a long week, will feel very different from exercising on a Monday morning after a full weekend of rest. Proper rest is sometimes the only cure for fatigue. According to recent research, the average person sleeps about two hours less per night than he or she did twenty years ago. Sound sleep is essential for effective exercise. Your body and its metabolism will also vary with the seasons. In winter, it takes more time to warm up the body whereas in the summer our bodies remain at higher temperatures. Eating habits also come into play. I find that my body behaves very differently after lunch. Joseph Pilates compared heavy eating immediately followed by sitting or lying down, as "overloading the firebox with coal and then closing the drafts to the furnace." In contrast, food is the fuel of your body and if your tank is empty you may find your performance suffers. Joseph suggested we expend our energies in proportion to the amount of fuel we consume. Balance is the key.

rolling back

Be patient and gentle with your spine until you feel that rolling becomes natural and you can return to the seated position with ease.

❗ CAUTION

If you have a tight lower back and struggle to come back up from the roll, use the alternative below to warm up the spine beforehand.

emphasis	mobility
visual cue	hedgehog
repeat	10 times

1 Sitting tall, lift from your center, imagining a taut string connecting the crown of your head to the ceiling. Bend your legs and place your feet together, flat on the floor. Place your hands on your shins and pull in your stomach muscles.

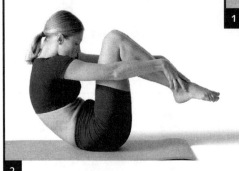

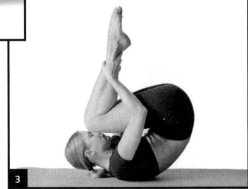

2 Taking a slow breath in, curl your pelvis and start the roll, with your chin near your chest and spine curled.

3 Gently roll back only as far as your shoulders. As you roll back up, with abs still contracted, begin to breathe out slowly. Complete the breath as you return to the seated position and lengthen your spine to the ceiling. Aim to make the roll as smooth as possible.

rolling back alternative

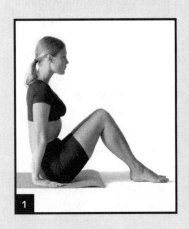

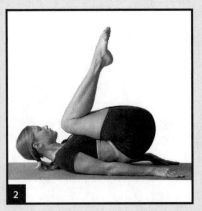

1 If you can't manage the above without straining, try this easier alternative. Use your hands as supports with palms down and close behind you.

2 Breathe in as you tilt the pelvis and roll back, using your arms to support your weight as much as needed while you roll up again.

62

one leg circle

This movement opens up the hip joint, increasing mobility.

⏸ CAUTION

If your hips move, you are taking the rotation too wide. You may find that each side has a different range of mobility. Limit your movement to the range allowed by the least flexible hip and keep the leg motion smooth. This will eventually restore balance to both hips.

emphasis	mobility
visual cue	clock
repeat	10 per leg

1 Lie relaxed and flat on the mat with your arms at your sides and palms down. Pull in your abs. Pointing your toes, stretch the left leg to the ceiling as far as possible without straining. Maintain a neutral spine (page 73).

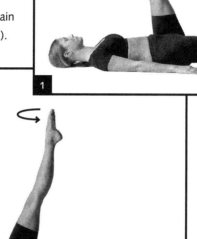

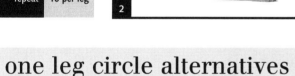

2 Rotate the left leg clockwise, using the hip joint as the center of the clock face. Always breathe in from 12 to 6 o'clock and breathe out from 6 to 12 o'clock. Repeat counterclockwise and then switch to your right leg.

one leg circle alternatives

ALTERNATIVE 1

Keep one leg bent at the knee, foot flat on the floor, to stabilize the body. This will decrease the range of rotation for the raised leg and make it easier to maintain a neutral spine. It may also help to imagine you are drawing a circle on the ceiling with your big toe. Breathe in and out, using the same clockwise rotation practiced in the previous movements.

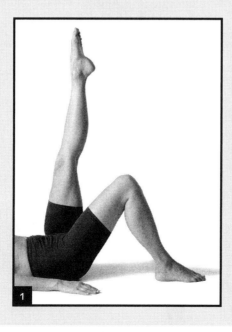

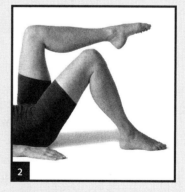

ALTERNATIVE 2

This time lower the raised leg to a 90° angle and draw the circle of the clock with your knee, stretching up from the hip.

the hundred

The hundred is used to strengthen the torso. You are challenging yourself to keep a neutral spine while counting to a hundred. Use your arms to count the rhythm and breathe in for five counts and out for five counts. Find a position that allows you to keep a neutral spine.

emphasis	strength
visual cue	steep slope
repeat	10 times

64

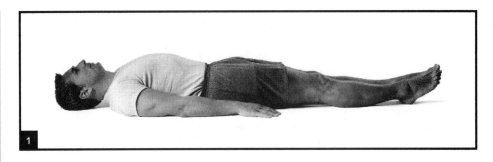

1 Lie on your back and check that your spine is neutral (page 73). Point your toes and lengthen your spine by pushing the top of your head away from you. Your shoulder blades should be pulled down your back.

2 Lift both legs up to a height where you still maintain a neutral spine. At the same time lift your head up off the floor. Imagine you are holding an orange under your chin. Your arms should be about six inches off the floor.

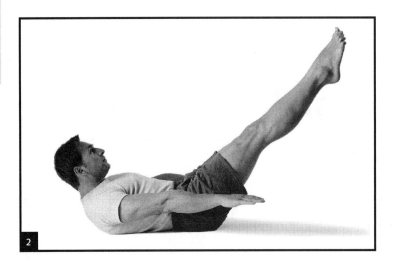

3 With a small movement, lower your straight arms about two inches off the floor and breathe in for five up-and-down beats and out for five beats. Repeat this ten times until you have completed a hundred beats.

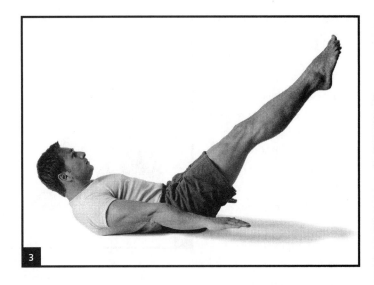

the hundred alternatives

1 Lower the intensity of the exercise by bending the knees, so shortening the weight you have to hold up. Remember, the longer your legs are stretched the more weight you must bear.

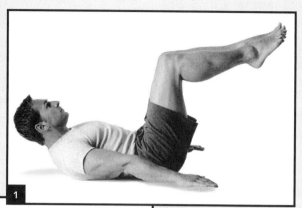

2 To further decrease the intensity and the weight lift, place the right leg on the floor for 50 counts and change to the left leg for the remaining 50 counts. Work between the variations to feel the difference on both sides of the body.

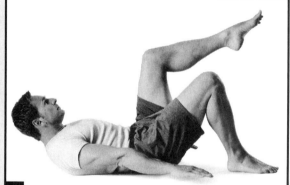

3 With both legs on the ground you have no weight to bear except that on your upper body. Try to maintain this position, always remembering that a neutral spine (see page 73) is your goal.

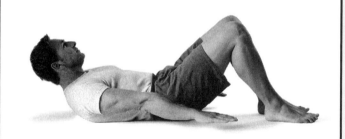

4 Keeping your head and shoulders down, maintain neutral spine as you breathe in for five counts and out for five. Do this 10 times. Use your arms to count the beats. If you want to start with two sets of 50 and then build to 100, keep your spine long and keep your shoulders pulled down your back.

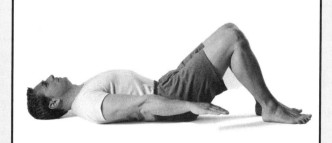

the seal

The second in the series of rolling exercises, this movement is used to create mobility and flexibility in the spine.

! CAUTION

If you find this too difficult, return to the basic rolling exercises where you may use your arms to support yourself.

emphasis	mobility
visual cue	rolling ball
repeat	10 times

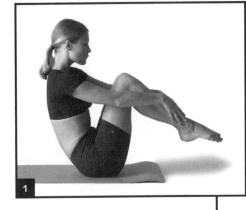

1 Take a balanced position holding your legs lightly. Lift the top of your head to the ceiling and contract your abs.

2 Breathe in as you roll back onto your shoulders. Stay in a tight ball. As you roll, imagine that you are imprinting your spine into the mat.

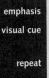

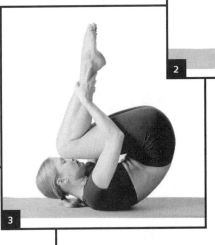

3 Breathe out as you come back up and return the roll to the seated position. Use the muscles at your center to power yourself back into the balanced position.

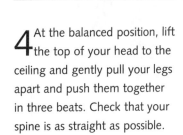

4 At the balanced position, lift the top of your head to the ceiling and gently pull your legs apart and push them together in three beats. Check that your spine is as straight as possible.

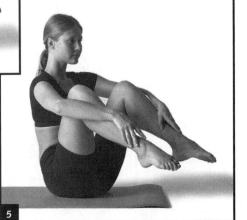

5 This beating of the feet adds to the balance period and also increases the strengthening element of the movement. Focus on your center and imagine it is initiating the pull. The strength for the balance position should also come from your center.

one leg stretch

1 Lifting your head and shoulders, hold your right leg gently and stretch the left leg away from you. The height of the leg is determined by the weight of your leg and the strength in your abs. Lift it higher if you feel your back arching.

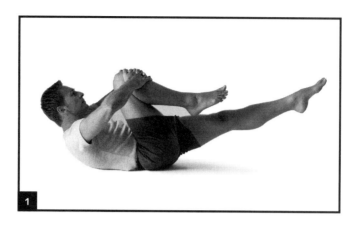

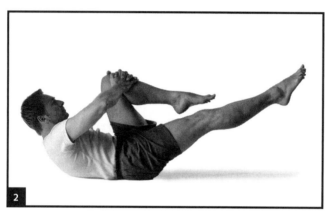

2 Slowly swap to the other leg. Keep the movement continuous and breathe in for two changes and breathe out for two changes. Keep your elbows lifted and your head in alignment. If you feel any stress in the neck, put your head and shoulders down.

one leg stretch alternatives

1 You can further decrease the intensity of this movement by lowering one leg to the floor and keeping your head and shoulders down. Hold your knee gently and check that your back is in neutral position (see page 73).

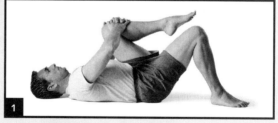

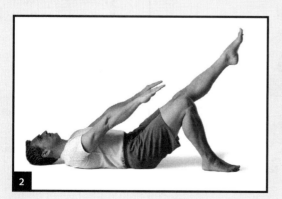

2 As you stretch your leg away from you, breathe out. Breathe in as it retracts toward your center. Try to ensure that your arms and legs are parallel and at the same angle. Repeat five times and then repeat with the other leg.

the saw

emphasis	mobility
visual cue	plane propellor
repeat	10 times

68

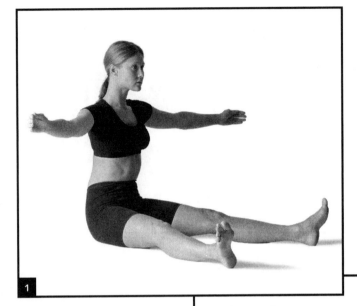

1 Sit with your legs hip-width apart and your feet flexed. Lift your arms either side of you. They should not be open too wide, just enough so that you can see them as you look forward. Lift your head up as though you are in a movie theater and trying to see over someone tall.

2 Breathe out and turn your body to the side. Keep your arms in line with your shoulders as you turn. Do not let them cross the body. Turn equally to the back and side keeping your hips facing firmly to the front.

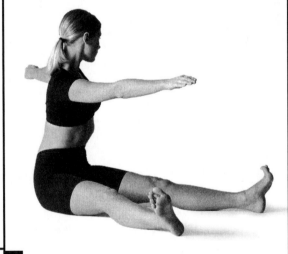

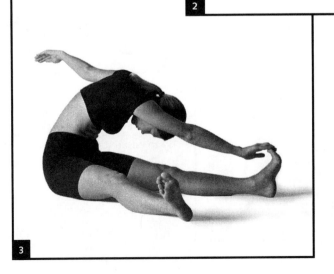

3 Continue to breathe out as you stretch over your leg to the point of tension. Imagine you have a large beach ball over your knee and that your are stretching over it. Keep your head down as you stretch. Breathe in as you come back to the center and repeat in the opposite direction on the other side.

shoulder bridge preparation

This movement is for opening and mobilizing the whole spine.

!CAUTION

Do not force this movement. Be very gentle with your spine. If you know you have a tightness in a certain area, then slow right down as you pass through it. Concentrate on gently coaxing your muscles into becoming flexible.

emphasis	mobility
visual cue	ski slope
repeat	10 times

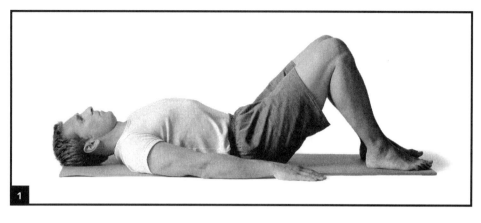

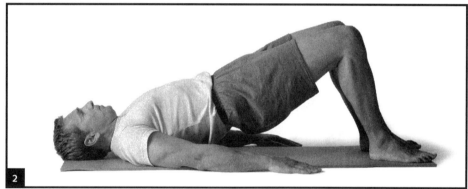

1 Lie on your back with your arms by your side. Think of the top of your head pulling you to one end of the room and your tailbone stretching to the other. Breathe in as a preparation, keeping your center strong.

2 Breathe out and start rolling up toward the ceiling leading with your tailbone, letting your vertebrae lift one by one from the mat. Lift your hips up taking them to the height where your body forms a slope, no higher.

3 At the top of the movement stretch your arms behind you and breathe in. As you breathe out start rolling down back to the mat as if laying a string of pearls on a piece of velvet. Visualize each vertebra as it touches the mat.

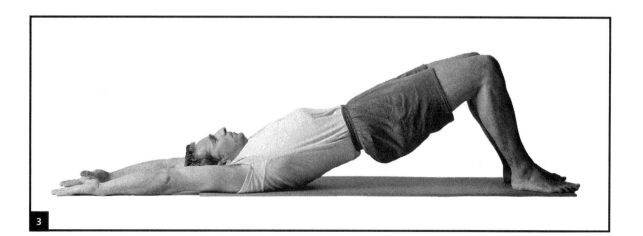

side kick

This is a stretch move that challenges you to keep your balance as you take your leg forward.

❚ CAUTION

Keep your shoulders stretched and do not allow your upper arm to move back. Do not lift your leg so far that you begin to lose your balance.

emphasis	strength
visual cue	side leap
repeat	10 times each side

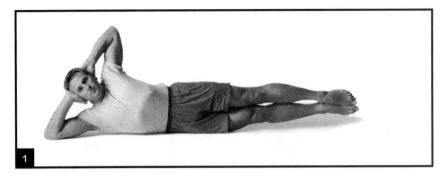

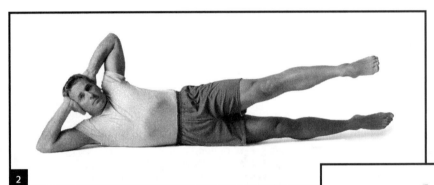

1 Lie on your side and check that your spine is in a horizontal line. Pull in your abs. Your hips should be stacked one on top of each other. Stretch your legs as you also pull your upper body away from your center.

2 Breathe out as you bring the top leg forward and breathe in as you slowly take it back. Find the range to keep control. Your strength is your center and your body works as a whole.

side kick alternatives

1 To reduce the balance and lower the intensity of this movement, lie down on your arm and place your upper arm in front of you. Check that your body is straight.

2 To further decrease the intensity of the movement, lift your torso on your elbow and place your upper arm behind your head. Check that you are lifting up off the floor with your upper body. You should feel no stress in your shoulders as you do this.

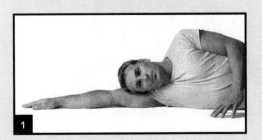

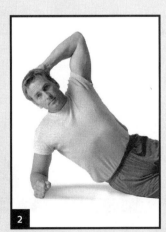

spine stretch

emphasis	mobility
visual cue	beach ball
repeat	10 times

1 Sit with your legs in front of you and apart, your hands on the floor between them. Flex your feet and pull up from your abs, lifting your head to the ceiling. Keep extending yourself. Do not reach the same point as you come up but try to accomplish a higher point. Also think about your shoulders stretching to the sides, as if opening up the body wider.

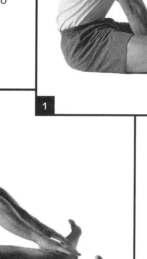

1

2 Breathe out as you round your back and stretch forward. Try imagining you are stretching over a large beach ball. Take it to the point of tension and then roll back up, stacking the vertebrae one by one. Do not stop at any point in this movement but keep it free and flowing.

2

spine stretch alternative

Bend your knees and lift your toes then carry out the movement described above. If your arms get tired, you can bend the arms to a Cossack position and let your hands touch your shoulders. Stretch your spine from the base, tilting from the floor. Try not to curl your back or crunch over your abs.

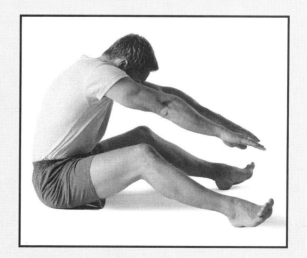

spine twist

This movement works on the mobility of the upper back.

❗ CAUTION

Do not think of this movement as a stretch. Think of it as a spine-rotating exercise in which you twist from side to side. Work gently on correcting any imbalances until the motion is smooth.

emphasis	mobility
visual cue	plane propellor
repeat	10 times

72

THE ESSENTIALS

1 Sit with your legs apart and your arms stretched out wide to the sides. Do not extend your arms too far, they should rest at right angles to your outstretched legs. Now pull in your abs and straighten and lift your head. Imagine, once again, that a hook at the top of your head is pulling you to the ceiling.

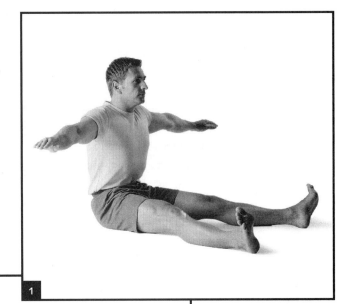

1

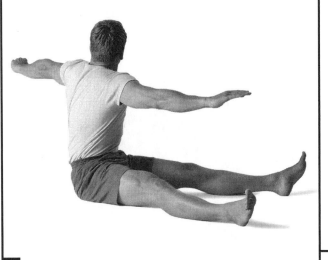

2

2 Breathe out as you turn to the side, keeping your head reaching to the ceiling and your hips facing to the front. When you reach the point of tension, try to relax the body a little further.

3 Breathe in as you come to the center and breathe out as you repeat the movement to the other side. Keep trying to take it a little further each time without forcing anything. If your arms get tired, you can cross your arms across your chest or bend your elbows so that your hands touch your shoulders.

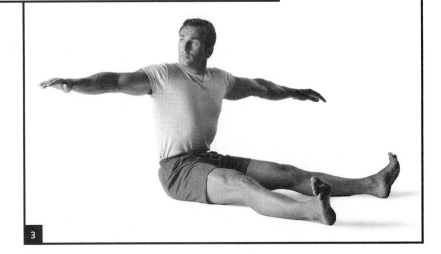

3

spine twist alternative

This variation can be used if you find it difficult to sit up straight with your legs spread in front of you.

! CAUTION

If you are tense in your shoulders then it is easy to tense them more as you turn. Bend your elbows and touch your shoulders.

Sit with your knees bent, feet touching. Your legs do not have to have to be held too closely together. If you feel them tensing, push them further away in front of you. Now do the exercise described left. Sitting on a book or towel will help you to straighten out and sit up properly.

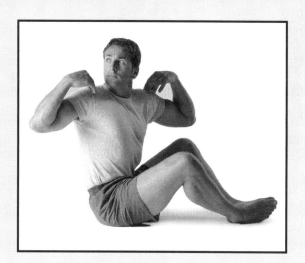

neutral spine

Many of the Pilates movements require you to maintain a "neutral spine." This is simply a term used to describe the natural curvature of your backbone. We all have three curves in our spine, the cervical (neck), the thoracic (upper back) and the lumbar (lower back). A correctly positioned spine should be S-shaped (although in reality the shape of your spine will be much softer and less pronounced than the curly letter S might imply). Bad posture makes us slump forward to form a C-shape.

Supine position

Explaining the idea of neutral spine is not always easy as it is not a fixed position. In order to find your own natural position try this easy exercise. Lie on your back on the floor with your knees bent. Gently push your back down to touch the floor (in aerobics this used to be called a "flat back"). If you were to stand up with your spine in this position you would be stooping over. Now take the body to the other end of the spectrum and gently arch your back. The neutral position is measured about half way between these two extremes. Simply let your back relax into its normal "supine" shape. Do not push your feet on the floor or tilt your pelvis up. Now put your hand under your back. You will find a space there. For some of us it is large and for others it is small. Everyone has a slightly different neutral position because we all come in slightly different shapes and sizes.

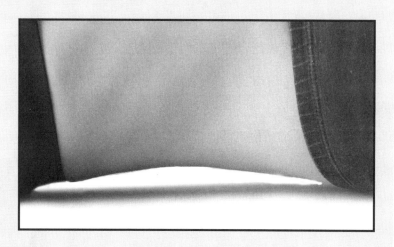

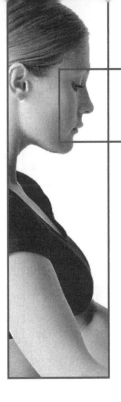

new challenges

After mastering some of the essential movements, try these more challenging and progressive ones. Listen to what your body tells you and only add them to your program when you feel ready and able. It is fine to challenge yourself but do not exceed the comfortable range of movement or try so hard that you lose control and begin to struggle.

the crab

Like all the rolling movements, the crab uses your body weight to stretch the spine. Aim to slow the movement down until it can be completed with control of your abdominals.

❗ CAUTION

Don't be surprised if you roll off to one side initially. This will decrease with time and practice.

emphasis	mobility
visual cue	crab
repeat	10 times

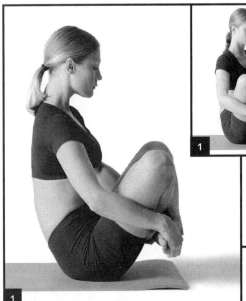

1 Use the same starting position as in rolling back (page 62). Cross your feet in front of you maintaining balance. Contracting your abs, lift your feet off the mat. Bring your arms around the legs and gently grasp the left foot with the right hand and the right foot with the left hand. Lift the feet slightly up toward your chest.

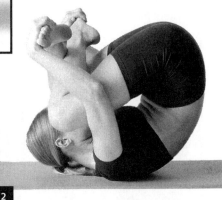

2 Initiate the roll by tilting the pelvis backwards. Breathe in on the roll down. Breathe out on the roll up, as you lengthen your body out. Remember to roll back only as far as your shoulders and to maintain control throughout. If this is hard, return to the seal.

double leg stretch

This movement is used to strengthen your abdominals and lower back. The weight of your legs and large circular motion of your arms challenge you to maintain a neutral spine throughout.

❗ CAUTION

If you begin to shake or are unable to maintain a neutral spine, raise your legs higher and decrease your arm movements. Otherwise try the alternatives below.

emphasis	**strength**
visual cue	**morning stretch**
repeat	**10 times**

1 Lay flat on the mat, contract your abs and maintain a neutral spine. Bring your knees in to your chest and place your hands on them.

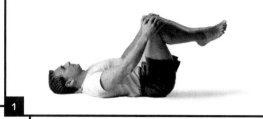

2 Breathe in, straighten your legs and arms to a 45° angle and raise your head and shoulders off the mat. Keep your chin and head in line with your arms and legs.

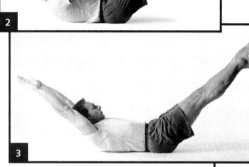

3 Without moving your legs, start the large continuous arm circles by stretching your arms back over your head to your ears.

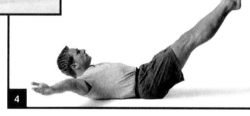

4 Without pausing, pull your arms out to the sides, completing the circle by returning them to the 45° angle and back to your knees.

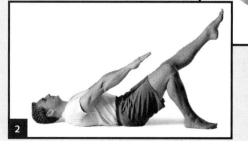

double leg stretch alternatives

These easier alternatives provide greater stability and allow a wider range of movement with the arms.

❗ CAUTION

If you continue to experience strain in these two positions, simply keep both knees bent and feet flat on the floor for the time being.

ALTERNATIVE 1
Take some strain off your lower back by bending one leg and placing your foot flat on the mat.

ALTERNATIVE 2
If you feel strain in your neck and shoulders, keep them on the mat while completing the arm circle.

rocker with open legs

This movement works on the mobility of the spine. With the legs lifted you are also building up your strength.

▋CAUTION

If you find the leg position in this movement too hard, try less intense movements such as basic rolling (p62) or the seal (p66).

emphasis	mobility
visual cue	rocking chair
repeat	10 times

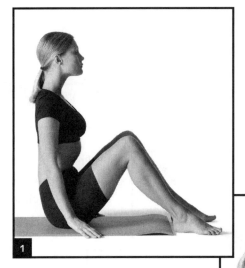

1 Sit with your legs in front of you, knees up and slightly apart. Lift up your head as though it is strung to the ceiling. Pull in your abs. Open your shoulders, rolling them well down your back.

2 Hold your ankles and lift your legs to a balanced position. Push your legs away from you as you lift your head to maintain a long spine.

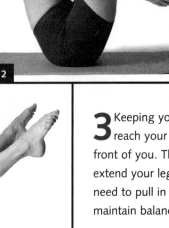

3 Keeping your balance, reach your legs out in front of you. The further you extend your legs the more you need to pull in your abs to maintain balance.

4 Breathe in as you roll back, keeping your legs the same distance from your body. Breathe out as you return to the balance position. Bend your knees slightly so you can touch your toes.

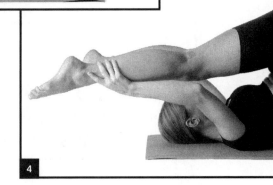

NEW CHALLENGES

shoulder bridge

This movement tests your core strength.

❗ **CAUTION**

Don't arch your back too much. Keep your shoulders, hips, and knees in a straight line.

emphasis	strength
visual cue	ship's mast
repeat	10 times each side

1 Lie on your back with your knees bent and feet hip-width apart. Stretch your arms down by your side and stretch your spine up toward your head.

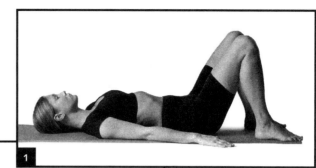

2 Breathe in as you roll your hips up toward the ceiling, peeling your spine from the mat vertebra by vertebra. Keep your abs pulled in. Only roll up as far as your shoulders.

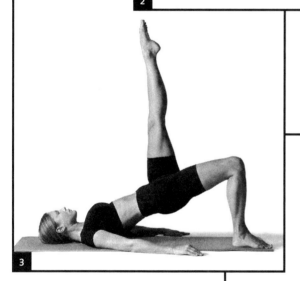

3 Breathe out as you unfold your left leg toward the ceiling, keeping your hips at the same height and not allowing them to drop. Use the strength in your center to hold you in place.

4 Breathe in as you bring your leg down again, pointing your toe away from you.

5 Try to touch the floor as you stretch the leg down. Breathe out as you lift the leg back to the ceiling. Breathe in as it touches the floor again. Slowly breathe out as you roll the spine back down, laying the vertebrae back onto the mat one by one.

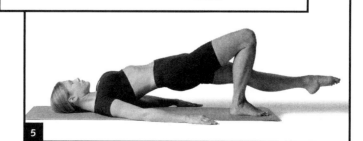

side bend

emphasis	strength
visual cue	leaning tower
repeat	10 times each side

1 Sit on your right hip with your right arm straight, resting your hand below your shoulder. Bend your left leg and place it in front of your right leg, which should be straight. Lift your head and tuck in your abs. Try to keep your hips forward so they are stacked one on top of the other.

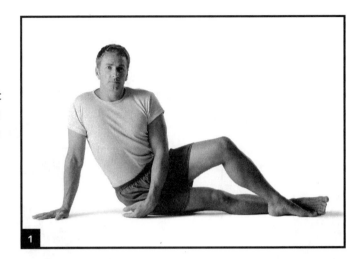

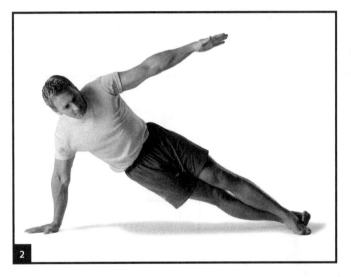

2 Breathe out as you push on your left foot and start lifting your body toward the ceiling. Reach out and up to the ceiling as your left arm draws a semicircle through the air along your side. Your strength is in your center, which pulls in to create the movement. Keep your spine long as you begin to lift.

3 Continue to stretch until you are fully extended. Breathe in as you slowly lower your body back to the starting position. Keep your speed the same when you move up and come down. Try to support yourself and keep your weight steady between each movement until you have completed the 10 repetitions.

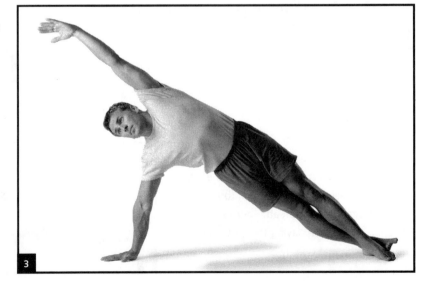

side bend alternatives

By lowering the movement you lower the degree of control needed to balance correctly.

❗ CAUTION

Keep your ribcage lifted up and don't let your shoulders sink. Don't place your weight onto your shoulders only.

ALTERNATIVE 1

1 Rest your body on your elbow, letting your hand reach forward in front of you. Lift your hand behind your head. Keep your abs tight.

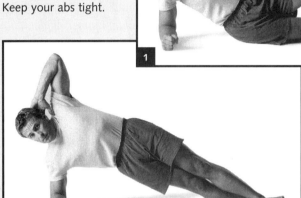

2 Push up as you breathe out and lift your hip to the ceiling. Keep your hips stacked and try not to let them move or roll forward.

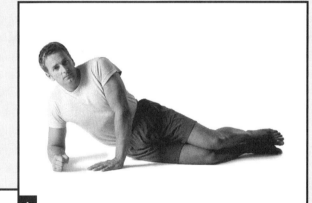

Lower the intensity by keeping your hand on the floor. and bending both knees.

❗ CAUTION

Keep any tension out of the region of your shoulders by sliding them down your back and mentally pinning them in place.

ALTERNATIVE 2

1 Keep your left hand on the floor as you rest on your right elbow. Bend both knees, keeping your knees and feet on top of each other. Don't let your hips roll forward.

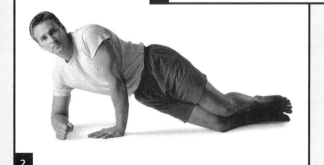

2 Breathe out as you lift your hips up off the floor and only lift them to a height where you can keep control. Breathe in as you lower yourself back down.

side-kick kneeling

80

NEW CHALLENGES

This movement is designed for strength. It challenges you to keep your torso in a neutral position as you use the weight of the leg swinging forward for balance.

❚ CAUTION

Do not try this if you have any history of problems with your knees.

emphasis	strength
visual cue	balancing scales
repeat	10 times each side

1 Kneel with your legs slightly apart and your arms stretched down by your side. Check that you are balanced in the center and your pelvis is relaxed in neutral. Lift your eyeline as if you are looking out over the horizon and pull up on your abs, checking that your back is still in neutral position.

1

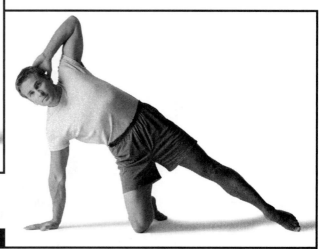

2

2 Move your weight out onto your right arm and make sure that you are evenly balanced on your arm and right leg. Point your toe and stretch the leg away from you, stretching your head and neck away in the opposite direction.

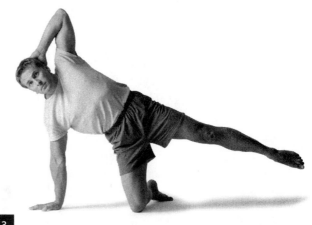

3

3 Pulling in your abs, lift your left leg to hip height.

4 Keeping your back in its neutral position, breathe out and bring your left leg forward at hip height. Your goal is to keep your back still as you move your leg. Breathe in as your leg comes back to align with your hip.

4

the teaser

1 Sit with your knees bent in front of you and hold your legs lightly. Pull up on your center as you straighten your head and pull yourself up toward the ceiling.

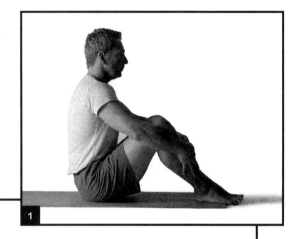

2 Breathe in and extend your legs, keeping a balanced position. Slowly lift your hands up toward your feet. Remember to keep your shoulders down your back.

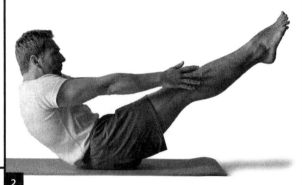

3 Feel your spine lifting off the mat, vertebra by vertebra. See how far you can extend yourself before you lose control of the movement.

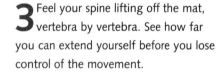

4 Breathe in as you let your body slowly roll down to the mat, and breathe out as you come back up to the balanced position. Keep the movement slow and smooth as you repeat it 10 times.

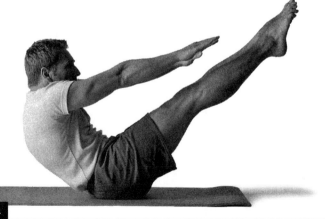

the jack knife

This is a strength maneuver that challenges you to lift the body up into a shoulder stand.

❚ CAUTION

Check that you have enough flexibility in the spine before you try this. By bending your knees during the movement you can reduce stress on the lower back.

emphasis	strength
visual cue	jack knife
repeat	10 times

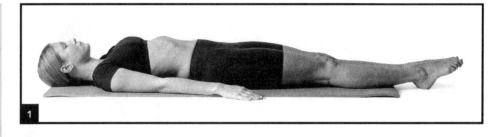

1 Lie flat on the floor with your arms down by your side. Stretch your head away from you.

2 Breathe out and lift your legs slowly up to the ceiling. Keep your feet above your face as they stretch upwards. Try not to use your arms too much: use your center as a powerhouse.

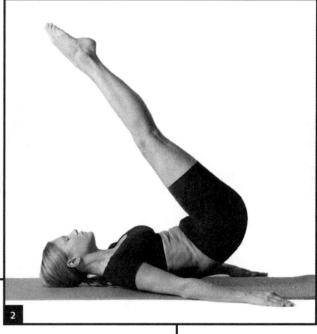

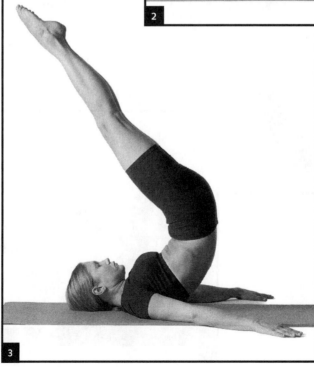

3 When you reach the highest point of your leg roll, slowly let your body come down to the floor again. It is not the stretch at the top of the movement that should be your goal but rather the journey getting there and coming back. The slower you do this movement, the more you will develop your strength.

hip twist

This is a strength movement that requires you to keep the torso still as you move the legs in a circle.

! CAUTION

The length of your legs makes a big difference to their weight—the longer the heavier. If you have long legs, you can bend your knees to lower the intensity of the movement to make it less strenuous.

emphasis	strength
visual cue	toe hoops
repeat	10 times

1 From a seated position breathe out and contract your abs as you lift your legs to a balanced position. Your hands are on the floor with your fingers pointing forward. Lift your head to the ceiling as you stretch your legs away from you.

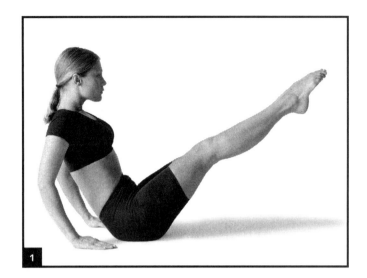

2 Take a breath in preparation and keep your body in a fixed position. Then circle your legs away from you as you breathe out. Focus on your abs being the control point from which the impetus for the circling begins.

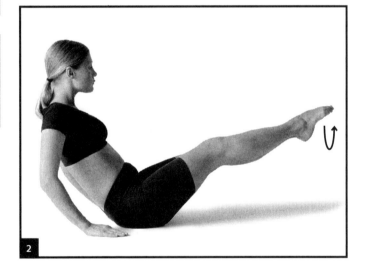

3 Complete the circle, holding the movement at the top and repeating it in the opposite direction. To lower the intensity you can lift the legs higher and bend your knees. You could also go back down onto your elbows. To really help you feel the effects of this exercise, get a friend to hold your shoulders still. Do not allow your shoulders to move as you perform the circles.

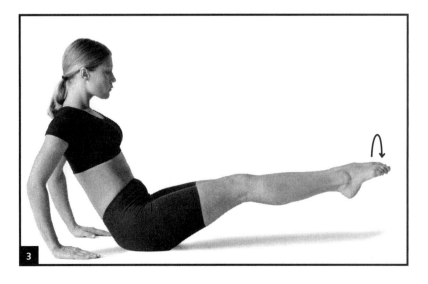

scissors

This is a strength movement that challenges you to stay balanced as you change legs.

█ CAUTION

Don't let your leg drop toward you. It will help if you keep focused on the leg that is the furthest away from you. Let this leg lead the slow "snipping" move.

emphasis	strength
visual cue	pair of scissors
repeat	10 times

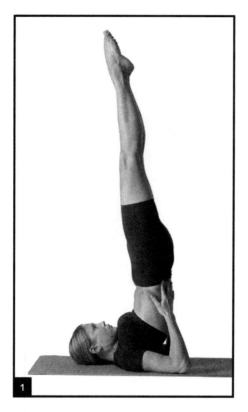

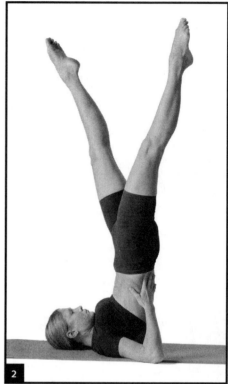

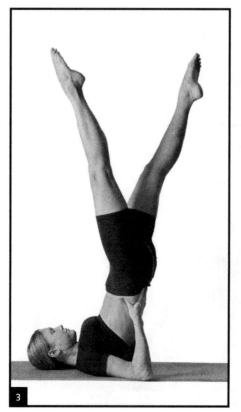

1 Lie on the floor, arms by your sides. Breathe out as you lift your body into a shoulder-stand position using the movement of a jack knife (page 82). Place your hands behind your back for support.

2 Breathe out as you open your legs an equal distance apart. Point your feet to the ceiling, stretching them as far as you can to lengthen the legs.

3 Breathe in as they close and change to the other side. Keep the movement consistent and slow as you find out how wide you can make each "snipping" move without your hips moving. Keep your hips pointing to the ceiling by using your abs to lift their weight off your elbows. Lengthen your neck and keep your shoulder blades pulled up, not crunched up.

scissors alternatives

The scissors can also be effective when it is performed closer to the floor. This will reduce the stress of gravity and make the movement easier to control. This alternative asks you to move your legs on a diagonal slope rather than on a vertical axis.

❚ CAUTION

Remember to keep your chin tucked in and begin the movement from your abs.

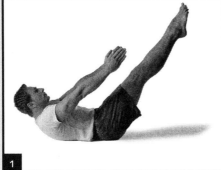

1 Lift up your legs until they form a diagonal slope. Slowly move your arms from your sides and point your fingers toward your toes.

2 Slowly move one leg down, keeping the other at the same height. Gently swap the legs around until you have completed the movement ten times.

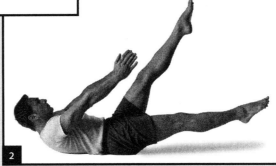

the rocker

This move is designed to strengthen your back by curling it backwards.

❚ CAUTION

This movement extends and pulls the muscles in the lower back. If you feel uncomfortable stresses in your lower back it is better not to lift so high from the floor.

emphasis	strength
visual cue	rocking chair
repeat	10 times

1 Lie face down and lift your legs holding onto your feet. Pull your abs in so that a piece of paper could pass under your navel. Stretch your legs and push your ears forward.

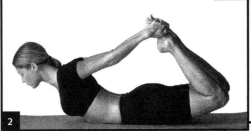

2 Keeping the strength in your center, lift your legs higher and breathe out. Take it to the point of tension that is most challenging.

3 Breathe in as you roll forward and breathe out as you roll back up. Keep the movement controlled, powering yourself from your center.

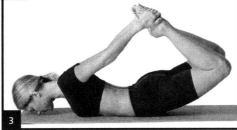

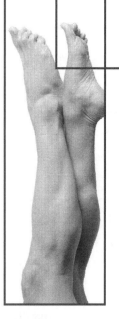

high intensity

These movements are the most challenging of all and will build strength and flexibility in equal measure. Only move on to these when you are confident that you are ready to do so. Remember all the vital elements of the Pilates technique as you attempt to perform them.

the boomerang

This movement is for mobility of the spine and uses your body weight and the weight of your legs.

⬛ CAUTION

This is the hardest of the rolling series. With your legs fully extended, there will be strain on your back muscles so, as always, it is extremely important to remember to warm up. If you feel too much strain, however, revert to the crab (page 74) or one of the other easier rolling series.

emphasis	mobility
visual cue	sling shot
repeat	10 times

1 Sit with your legs in front of you, your right leg crossed on top of your left. Reach your legs forward and pull in your abs. Keep your head upright and let your arms rest down by your sides. Move your shoulders so that they are open and rest down your back.

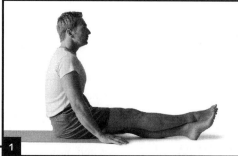

2 Lean your body forward and let your arms reach behind you. Fix the position of your body as you reach your point of tension.

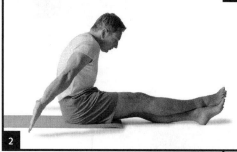

3 Breathe in as you roll back up onto your shoulders. Keep your legs straight and use your arms as stabilizers. Breathe out as you come back up to the forward position. Control your legs as they gently touch the ground in front of you. Keep the movement smooth.

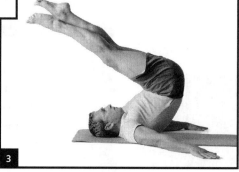

neck pull

This movement builds strength and tests your ability to lift the body from the floor.

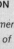 **CAUTION**

This movement uses the weight of the arms to add intensity to the movement. It also adds intensity to the back. If you feel stress, then perform a lower version.

emphasis	strength
visual cue	folding over
repeat	10 times

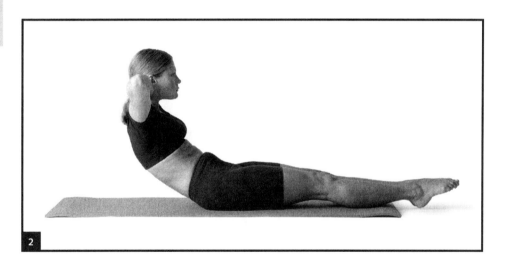

1 Lie on the floor with your arms behind your head and your fingers clasped. Stretch your legs out straight with your toes pointing away from you. Check that your back is in neutral position and you are pulling in on your center.

2 Slowly roll forward and peel your back off the floor as you breathe out. Keep the movement very smooth and slow; if you feel any strain in your back let your arms down. Pull in and up on your abs and bend your knees.

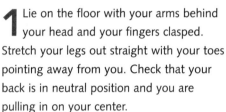

3 Stretch forward to the point of tension and then, without stopping, roll back down, laying your vertebrae onto the mat one by one. Try to be aware of each disc and feel each vertebra imprint into your mat, imagining that the mat is made out of soft putty.

control balance

This is the hardest of all of the movements because your arms are not stabilizing you. It builds strength and challenges you to keep your balance while moving your legs.

❗ CAUTION

Make sure you have enough flexibility to perform this under exercise with enough control.

emphasis	strength
visual cue	sprung coil
repeat	10 times

HIGH INTENSITY

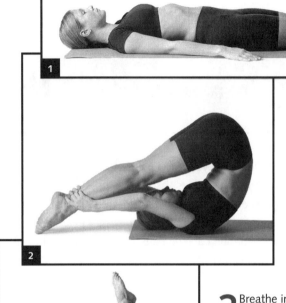

1 Lie on the floor with your back in a neutral position, your legs straight and your arms down by your sides.

2 Breathe out as you lift your legs slowly over your head until they touch the floor. Grab on to your ankles as you exhale.

3 Breathe in as you reach your right leg up to the ceiling, lengthening your body along both the raised and lowered legs. Work from your powerhouse center to maintain balance.

4 Breathe out as you slowly change to the other leg without stopping, keeping the movement continuous as you pass through each point of the move.

5 After you have finished the series, breathe in and slowly lower the leg back down, breathing in so that both legs are above your head. Then roll back down to the mat, adopting the original position as you breathe out.

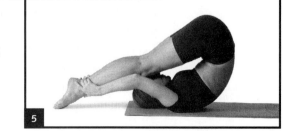

leg pull supine

This movement builds strength as you test your abs to keep your hips aloft while you move your legs.

! CAUTION

Keep your body weight off your shoulders by pulling your shoulder blades down your back and keeping your neck stretched long.

emphasis	strength
visual cue	pair of scissors
repeat	10 times

1 Start in a sitting position with your legs straight in front of you. Place your hands on the floor, shoulder-width apart, with your fingers pointing toward your knees. Keep the top of your head lifted up toward the ceiling. Pull your abs in and pull your shoulders down your back.

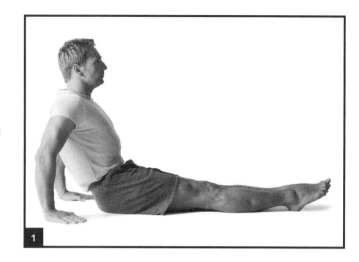

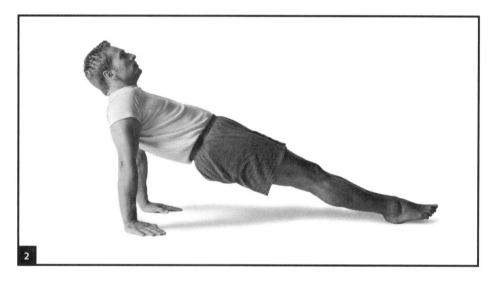

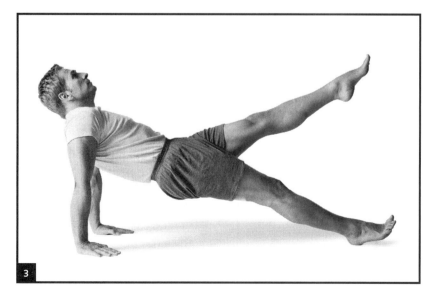

2 Breathe in as you raise your hips to the ceiling, making a straight line from your shoulders through your hips and ankles.

3 Breathe out as you raise your left leg to the ceiling, keeping your hips in a fixed position. Focus on your center of power to lift your legs. Breathe in as you lower one leg and change to the other. Repeat 10 times on each leg before slowly lowering it. Keep the flow continuous as you change legs.

the corkscrew

This movement builds strength and demands that you control the move even as you spin off balance.

▌CAUTION

It is very important that before you challenge yourself with an off-balance move you have built up enough strength at your center.

emphasis	strength
visual cue	side
	twist
repeat	10 times

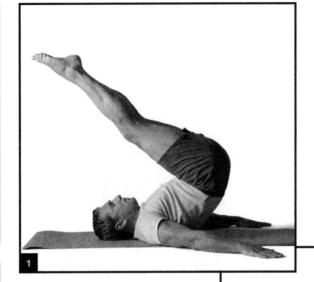

1 Lie flat on the floor with your arms by your sides. Breathe out as you slowly raise your legs and torso up and over your head, letting your toes touch the floor. Slowly peel your back off the floor. Keep your arms down by your side to help you up off the floor; check that your shoulders are pulled down your back. Breathe in when you reach the top point of the movement.

2 Breathe out and let your legs start drawing a semicircle together. Start with a small circle to keep control, then try to find the point where you threaten to lose control. Feel the one side of your spine laying down on the floor as you complete the semicircle.

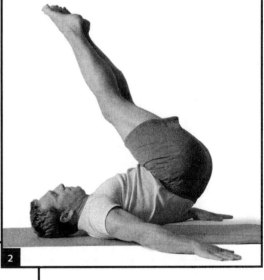

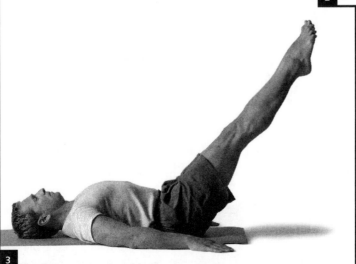

3 As your tailbone touches the floor slowly breathe in and repeat the movement, lifting your legs up and over your head. This time, take the semicircle to the other side. Work evenly on each side and remember—the slower the movement, especially on the downward phase, the more strength you are building. Keep your actions continuous, flowing evenly.

rollover

1 Lie with your arms slightly out to the side and your feet pointing away from you. Slowly lift your legs from the ground and up over your head. Keep your toes pointed. Feel each vertebra lift up from the mat as you bring your legs further over the rest of your body.

2 Keep moving your legs until your feet gently touch the floor behind your head. Use your arms to keep control and maintain balance.

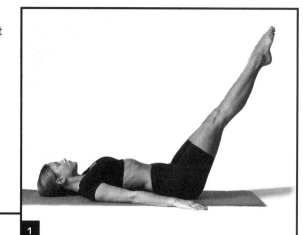

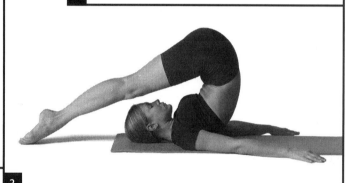

3 Continue the movement and bring your legs back up over your head. Try to keep the action continuous.

4 When your legs have come through the cycle and are back in position, open your legs until your toes reach beyond your hands. Do not attempt to open them too wide. Bring them together and begin the movement again.

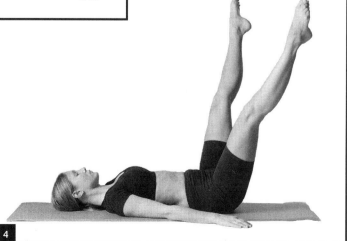

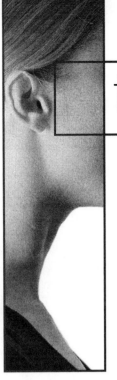

tips to remember

Nearly all the Pilates movements require you to adopt some positions that may at first feel uncomfortable. Here, I've set out the best ways to think about how you should hold your body during the exercises. You need to assume the right positions in order to complete the movements correctly and to ensure that you do not inadvertently injure yourself.

abdominals

It is important to make sure you are breathing correctly when exercising your abdominal muscles. It is usual to find yourself breathing in when you pull in your abs and breathing out when your belly bulges. However, you need to do the opposite of this. Breathe out as you pull in your navel and tuck in your abdominal muscles.

When I talk about "your center" I am referring to the area that lies between your ribs and your hips. For many people, the abdominal muscles are the most neglected area of their bodies. Flabby bellies are testament to our neglect of this region. Simply tucking in the abs can often cause pain or short breath. Yet Joseph Pilates nicknamed the abdominal area "the powerhouse" precisely because our entire body strength originates at our center. The abdominals act as a second spine in that they support the back and help to keep us erect. The muscles comprise of various layers: the rectus abdominals, the internal and external obliques and the traversus abdominals. Some of the Pilates movements focus on the latter which are positioned around your midriff, much where a belt would lie on a pair of low-slung, hipster trousers. Through Pilates you will become more aware of your abs.

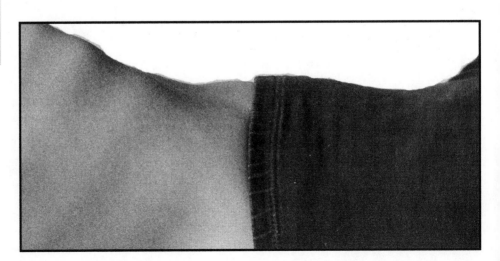

neck

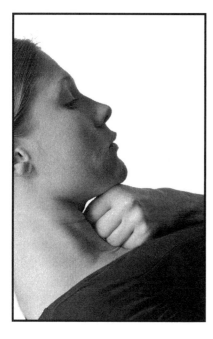

It is important for us to build the neck strength as the neck supports the weight of the head. On average one head weighs between 14 and 18 lbs. Many Pilates exercises expect us to be able to carry this weight, but like any strengthening process, it can take time. If you feel at any point that there is too much stress on your neck, then put your hands behind your head. It is very important that your head is in alignment with the rest of your body when you perform the movements. I have found the easiest way to check this is to put my fist between my chin and chest so that my head rests just on top of it. Another good check is to imagine that you are holding an orange under your chin. This stops you jutting your chin forward and straining your neck muscles or jamming your chin onto your chest. Use these methods to check that you are performing the movements correctly. If you have a stiff neck in the morning after doing these movements then you have pushed yourself a little too much. The next time you practice, put your arms back to support your head much sooner.

shoulders

In all of the movements, your shoulder muscles should be pulled well down your back. When we try to use our shoulders in strength movements, it is normal to find that they have a tendency to rise up our backs and hunch up around the neck. Stand up straight and feel the position in which ideally they should remain. I like to think of them as two plates that I need to slide down my back. When you put your shoulders in position down your back, your chest will automatically push forward and out and you will find that your whole appearance and look changes. Try to maintain this shoulder position when you are sitting and standing. At the beginning you will have to think constantly about adjusting your shoulders but, with time, you will find you can adopt this pose more easily and more naturally.

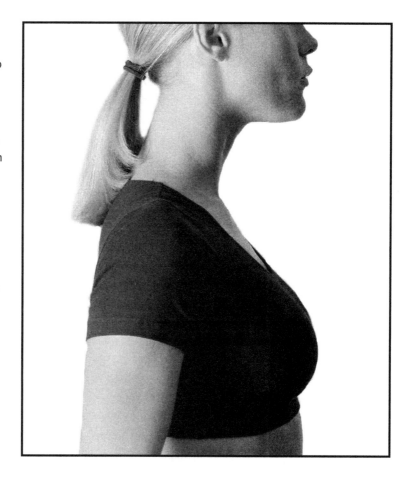

glossary

Abdominal muscles (abs): the muscles layered across the midriff that lie across each other at various angles. There are four types: the rectus abdominals, internal obliques, external obliques and transversus abdominals.

Aerobic exercise: any sustained activity that works the heart and lungs, increasing the amount of oxygen in the blood.

Alignment: arrangement in a straight line.

Cardiovascular: relating to the heart or the blood vessels.

Centering movements: the Pilates exercises that work the center of the body, abdominals and back.

Contrology: the name given by Joseph Pilates to his exercise method, which he defined as "the science and art of coordinated body–mind–spirit development through natural movements under strict control of the will."

Core exercises: the Pilates movements that concentrate on strengthening the abdominal and back muscles.

Crunching: sit-ups where the abdominals are not engaged so much as squeezed together, shortening the space between the hips and ribcage.

C-shape: the shape of the spine when the body is slumped over and bent due to bad posture.

Elongation: lengthening of the muscle. Leaner muscles develop from stretching the muscle rather than bulking it up.

Hidden stress: when muscle groups compensate for an injury or difficulty by using larger muscles to protect weaker ones.

Hunching: result of neck and shoulder tension within the trapezius muscles. Muscles here can tense up in an automatic defensive reaction.

Hyperextension: extending further than 180 degrees. This occurs when the muscles tense up and the elbows or knees lock, resulting in a reverse bending.

Imprinting: gently pushing each vertebra into the mat, as though it were leaving an indentation.

Lumbar curve: the bend of the spine at the small of the back.

Overloading: point where the effort required by a muscle to withstand an applied weight is too great. The tissue may tear or rupture as a result.

Powerhouse: The name that Joseph Pilates gave to the abdominal area, found between our ribcage and hips. Pilates exercises work this area in order to create a stronger, more balanced lower back.

Prone: lying face down.

Resistance: an opposing force that pulls in the direction opposite to the one created by your muscle.

Rolling: exercises where the spine rolls over the mat, one vertebra at a time.

Soft knees: holding the knees relaxed and slightly bent, rather than locked.

Supine: lying down on the back.

Tendon: elastic linking tissue that connects bone to muscle.

Tripod position: where the feet support the body weight by distributing it evenly over three points: the ball of the foot, the middle of the heel and the outside edge of the foot, near the little toe.

Vertebra: one of the bony segments that make up the spinal column.

Visualization: use of mental imagery to aid the accomplishment of physical tasks—an important element of the Pilates technique that helps the mind more effectively control the body.

index

acknowledgements

I would like to thank my mother and family for being so supportive of me, a boy from Scunthorpe, a Northern steelworks town, who wanted to go to dance school. (Thanks, John Travolta, for making it OK for men to dance.) I must also sincerely thank my mentor and teacher Alan Herdman, who first inspired me to pursue Pilates as a career, and the many other Pilates teachers who have shared their knowledge with me. Thanks to my friend David, who told me I wasn't crazy when I wanted to open my own studio at Pineapple when no one had ever heard of Pilates. To my friends at Houston Ballet who made me feel like the city was my second home. To Malcolm, for all his support and encouragement through this incredible last year. To all at Mitchell Beazley publishers, especially Rachael, Emma, Mary, Frances and Kenny for their sweet demeanors and cool heads as deadlines approached. And finally, I thank all those who have attended my classes all over the world over the years. It's been great!